About the Author

Art is a graduate of the University of Southern California School of Pharmacy. He has had specialized clinical experience in professional, community, hospital and geriatric pharmacy, before turning his interests to a more natural philosophy. He is one of the first modern trained pharmacists to become an avid supporter of preventative and complimentary medicine.

Art has his own consulting company, and is involved in numerous ventures in the nutritional supplement and health alternative industry. His activities include, field educational programs, product development, marketing, consumer and professional seminars, publishing, and business opportunity consultation.

When not on the road or on a trail, Art resides in a village-like community, with his attractive wife Janet, on beautiful Monterey Bay in California. His hobbies are mountaineering and "catch and release" fly-fishing.

Pharmacist's Guide to

Medicinal Herbs

By

Dr. Arthur M. Presser

Smart Publications
PO Box 4667
Petaluma, CA 94955

707.763.3944 (Fax)
www.smart-publications.com

PHARMACIST'S GUIDE TO MEDICINAL HERBS

By Dr. Arthur M. Presser

Published by:
Smart Publications™
PO Box 4667
Petaluma, CA 94955

Fax: 707 763 3944
www.smart-publications.com

Copyright 2000 by Smart Publications™

Library of Congress Catalog Card Number: 99-66309
First Printing 2000
Printed in the United States of America
First Edition

ISBN: 1-890572-13-6 $14.95   Softcover

Warning - Disclaimer

Dedication

To my wife and soul mate, Janet, whose unending support allowed me to overcome the obstacles standing in the way of this project's completion.

Disclaimer

The author has written this book, and the publisher has published this book with the intent to provide educational material. It is not intended to serve as a prescription, and under no circumstances to be considered a substitute for the advise of your medical doctor. Every effort has been made to make this book as accurate as possible, given the dynamic nature of the subject matter. This book is sold with the understanding that neither the publisher nor author are liable for any erroneous belief or misuse of the information provided. The author and publisher disclaim any responsibility or liability to any person or entity with respect to any loss, injury, or damage caused or alleged to be caused, directly or indirectly, by the information contained in this book.

Forward

One need not look far to see the evidence that the herbal revolution is firmly taking hold in mainstream America. Once relegated to the shelves of health food stores, mail order catalogs, and multi-level marketing salespeople, herbal products now are sold in supermarkets, drugstores, and large mass market retailers, as well as convenience stores, gyms and spas, the internet, offices of conventional healthcare practitioners, and almost anyplace where consumer goods are sold.

A recent survey by *Prevention* magazine discovered that as many as 48 percent of American adults have used an herbal product in the past year, with 24 percent using them regularly. The reasons are fairly obvious: to ensure good health (75%), improve energy (61%), prevent or treat colds and flu (58%), improve memory (43%), reduce anxiety (41%), ease depression (35%), and prevent or treat serious illnesses (29%).

What's more, 36 percent of these consumers use herbal remedies instead of prescription drugs, and 31 percent use them *with* prescription drugs, while almost half (48%) use them instead of over-the-counter drugs or with OTC's (30%). It doesn't take a rocket scientist to figure out what could happen here: it is almost inevitable that some herb-drug interactions are bound to occur. Some of these are predictable, while some will constitute new information for health authorities to *kvetch* about.

Obviously, the rise in herbal usage presents new opportunities for consumers, as well as some potential risks. Like all therapeutically active substances, herbs should be used appropriately and responsibly. However, until only a very few years ago, it was most difficult for consumers and lay people to find authoritative, reliable information on how to use herbs in a responsible manner. Further, it was difficult to find a physician or pharmacist who knew anything about these products; there was little or no training in medical and pharmacy schools in herbal medicines. Most of the conventionally trained healthcare professionals I know have begun to develop their herbal knowledge *after* they graduated from medical or pharmacy school.

That's why someone like Dr. Art Presser is so refreshing. In my experience, he was one of the first conventionally trained pharmacists (actually, a Pharm.D., a doctorate in pharmacy, a course of study that requires an extra year more than most registered pharmacists take) who I have met who was on the herbal bandwagon before the train had left the station. Art has been studying herbs for years. He is one of the early birds in his profession, a conventionally trained professional who very early recognized that there is considerable value and benefit in the world of botanical medicine.

It is ironic that we make so much to do about the advent of herbal products in the pharmacies today – ironic because only a few years ago, back in the 1930s and earlier, that herbal products were found in drugstores everywhere across the U.S. Without going into a history lesson, suffice it to say that herbs were dropped from official status in the United States Pharmacopoeia in the 1930s, not because they were found to be unsafe or ineffective (this was never done), but because they fell by the wayside due to lack of use. The pharmacy and medical professions were becoming seduced by the much more dramatically acting new drugs of the day, the sulfa drugs and related pharmaceutical advances. Herbs were simply old medicines– to many, old but very reliable – but they could not compete with the new medicines, for a variety of reasons that are not worthy of discussion here.

Herbs fell away from the pharmacies, only to reappear a few decades later in the health food stores of the 1950s and 1960s. We all know what happened next: the market began a steady increase in the 1970s and 1980s, culminating in the boom we have witnessed in the past five years. During this boom, herbs have gone full circle, back on the shelves of the pharmacies.

It is fitting that pharmacists take on the role of helping to educate the public about the benefits and potential risks of herbs. Pharmacists are playing an increasingly significant position in patient care, and are often the only source of professional information for many patients. (It doesn't cost anything to walk up to the pharmacist at the grocery store and ask her or him a health-related question that might include something about herbs! There's no doctor's office visit, no fee, and no time away from work, etc.) At present, approximately 23 percent of herb users claim to get some of their information from their pharmacist. Who knows? This figure could be even higher. (Figures don't lie, but liars figure, as the saying goes.)

This book is a gratifying and welcome entry into the herbal literature. Not only does Dr. Presser draw from a vast scope of scientific research for this book, he writes in a tone that is credible and authoritative and yet at the same time accessible and witty. It provides lots of good information in an accessible style. Whether you are a consumer or health professional, you will enjoy a new perspective on the world of herbs through the experience and mindset of a recovered pharmacist.

—Mark Blumenthal
Founder and Executive Director, American Botanical Council
Editor, *HerbalGram*
Senior Editor, *The Complete German Commission E Monographs: Therapeutic Guide to Herbal Medicines*
Adjunct Associate Professor of Medicinal Chemistry, College of Pharmacy, University of Texas at Austin

Contents

Contents Continued......

Introduction

Botanists have currently identified about 250,000 different plant species, of which 13,000 have been used as plant medicines some-where in the world at some time in history. Of these 13,000, one thousand species are frequently used as plant remedies. And of this one thousand, about one-half are commercially available in the United States. Of this 500, we will be reviewing 50 botanical medicines in the following pages. This is hardly a comprehensive or complete materia medica—a scientific study of medicinal drugs and their sources, preparation, and use—and it is not intended to be. My intention is to help familiarize you with some of the most commonly used herbs on today's market, in addition to some very interesting ones, not com-monly used, yet. And perhaps in the process of learning about and using the first 50 herbs, you will develop a way of looking at the next 50, or 150, or 950. What are the stories behind the plant? What were its historical, traditional, or folkloric uses? What are its modern uses, and how are they related to its traditional uses? Has modern medicine finally validated primitive or ancient cultures' methods of healing, or has it improved on them?

I have tried to make this book approachable for everybody. I believe if you read it from cover to cover, you will be entertained and will learn a lot about many of today's most popular botanicals. After you are through, put it on your bookshelf and use it as reference book.

I have also included some material appropriate for health professionals and those more inclined to be interested in chemicals, mechanisms of action, and theories. This information can be found under the sub-heading "Science." The truth be known, I even tried to keep this uncomplicated. However, if in your opinion I did not succeed or if this is not your cup of tea, skip over this material. Trust me, you won't be missing anything essential for appropriately using this book. You will still get everything that is practical.

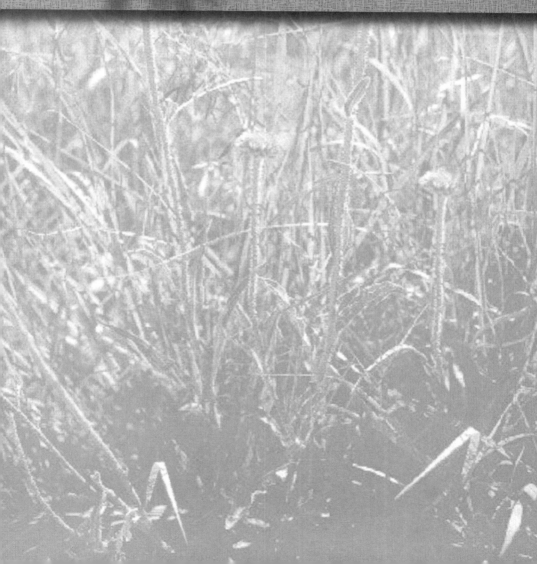

Part One

Herbology 101

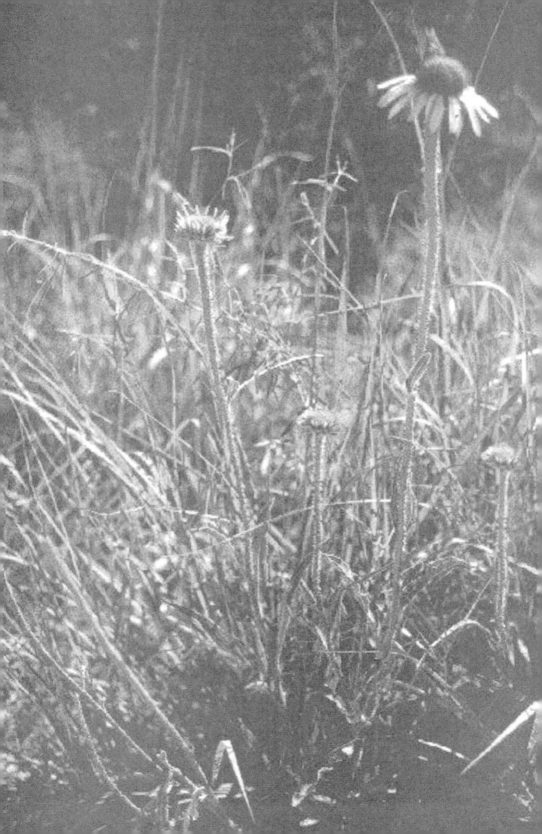

A Brief History of Botanical Medicine

From the beginning

A study of the history of herbal medicine is a study of civilization itself. It starts at the beginning and will probably end at the end. The use of herbs as medicines started in prehistoric times when man shared the earth with other animals and Nature. Man probably observed the animals around him and noticed that some of the carnivores would eat plants, instead of just a steady diet of themselves. Early man probably tried it, figured it wasn't all that bad, and then turned around and invented salad dressing.

Early man may have heeded which plants the animals avoided. And he may not have. But it probably didn't take too many companions keeling over dead around him to figure out that some plants were not to be eaten. He probably also noticed that some plants exerted various physiological effects on the body. I am sure our forbears took note and figured that at some time, they might be able to use that plant to produce that effect, rather than merely as food.

For example, maybe they ate a plant and found that it had a laxative effect. Then weeks later, when they overindulged on too many dinosaurs and were a little bound up, they remembered the antidote and went on an herb walk. The following winter when the problem returned, and the plant wasn't there, they must have really missed it. So, when spring brought the neighborhood back up to par, they said, "Hey, what if I cut up this plant and dry it in the sun? I'll wrap it in some Saran® wrap and tuck it away until I need it again." I think this is the way herbal medicine began.

At some point, the clan member with the most knowledge of Nature probably became the shaman or medicine man. His job was to develop techniques to quell adverse spirits, administer medicines, and bring the body back into harmony with the universe. These jobs are still available in the wilds of South America, Asia and Africa, if you're interested. And, I use the term "wild" very loosely, as I make many trips to Los Angeles and New York every year.

Herbal knowledge was verbally handed down from father to son, from family to family, from village to village, and from shaman to apprentice. This is because the Bic® and yellow pad were yet to come.

In Barbara Griggs' great book on the history of Western herbal medicine, *Green Pharmacy*, she reports on the excavation of a 60,000-year-old Neanderthal man's gravesite in Iraq. Thickly scattered in the dirt around his bones were the remnants of eight plants, seven of which are still used medicinally by the locals. Three are mainstream herbs used today, namely marshmallow, yarrow (one of this book's entries), and ephedra, (another entry and one of the world's most picked on botanicals).

Fast-forwarding 55,000 years, we stop at our oldest recognized ancient civilizations, the Chinese, Indian, and Egyptian. Now we have the ability to document and communicate over larger areas. Herbal books, called Herbals, or Materia Medicas from the Greek words meaning a list of medical materials, are beginning to be written. Herbal medicine is beginning to become a discipline.

Traditional Chinese Medicine

Chinese Herbal Medicine (CHM) is a branch of a larger medical system called Traditional Chinese Medicine (TCM). It is the oldest, most complete, safest, and perhaps most effective system of healthcare in the world. For more than 5,000 years, CHM has been the primary means of promoting health and longevity in the planet's longest ongoing civilization.

TCM is the sum of more than 5,000 years of wisdom. It is believed to have its origins in the toils of the legendary emperor Shen Nung (circa 3494 BC). He was fascinated with plants and their effects on the body, and tested many on himself. He also planted the seeds of the theory of opposing forces, which was later established as the "yin" and "yang" complements of Nature.

The old yin-yang
According to TCM, yin and yang are the two basic and opposing

principles of balance. Yin and yang are basic to Nature itself. They are opposing forces but, at the same time, are complementary, like summer and winter, day and night. They are contrary, but co-dependent. The Chinese believe that health can be attained, and maintained, by keeping the forces of yin and yang balanced.

Yin nurtures, preserves and forms life; yang dynamically generates and activates life.
The yin principle represents femininity, cold, water, and darkness. Yang represents masculinity, heat, fire and sun. Yin is for expansion, diffusion, lightness, fragility, and moisture. Yang is for contraction, fusion, heaviness, hardness, and dryness. When in balance, the opposing forces of yin and yang give rise to the dynamic wholeness that is health.

It was Shen Nung's feeling that the primary duty of the health care professional was to keep these opposing forces in harmony within the patient, and to restore equilibrium using either up-regulation or down-regulation of whichever force was out of balance as necessary. In fact, in time, this philosophical approach to disease prevention became such a trademark of TCM that doctors were often only paid when their patients were healthy. I wonder what that would do Western medicine?

Influence of Taoism
During the next 2,000 years, the era of the Shang Dynasty, the practice and theories of TCM were further developed by reclusive wise men intent on achieving immortality. Obviously, as they are not still with us, they never found their "Elixir of Life, but from their search evolved an acute insight into how the energies of plants, along with diet, exercise, and breathing were interrelated with the body's energy and health. This insight lead to the philosophy of Taoism, which further nurtured the basic principles of TCM. Taoism as a school of thought considers such standards as energy systems, sensations, and constant life changes and their interrelatedness to being.

It was the early Taoist philosophers who identified Chi (or Qi) as a vital force. Chi, the life-force in all living things, circulates through the body along energy lines called meridians. Sickness is believed to occur when an imbalance or congestion of this energy prevents its free flow or causes this life energy to flow against its natural direction. Acupuncture, herbal remedies, dietary considerations, and lifestyle changes are implemented to harmonize the flow of Chi, coaxing it back into the direction of wellness. According to the Taoists, to maintain the free flow of Chi is to achieve physical longevity and spiritual power.

During the Shang dynasty, the Yellow Emperor Huang Di authored the *Nei Ching*, the *Yellow Emperor's Classic of Medicine*, a monumental work on Chinese medical theory, herbalism, and acupuncture, and considered the principles of internal medicine. Most of ancient Chinese medical literature is founded on the *Nei Ching*, which is still regarded as a great authority.

Breaking from its shamanistic roots
By 1,500 BC, TCM had made its way into mainstream Chinese life. Archeological studies from that period have revealed a deep understanding of disease, diagnosis and treatment displayed by the healers of that era. As the culture thrived through the ensuing centuries, TCM became a more sophisticated discipline. By the end of the Han dynasty (circa 220 AD), the foundation of the Holy Grail of Chinese medicine, the Chinese Herbal Pharmacopeia, was firmly in place. From this time forward, the principles of TCM have only been refined, with no need for revolutionary discoveries.

Tang to Song to Ming, triple play
During the Tang, Song, and Ming dynasties, a period spanning over 2,000 years, TCM underwent scientific institutionalization. A system of medical schools was founded, standards of medical practice were developed, and herbal formulae were standardized. TCM moved away from Taoism and became more closely aligned with Confucianism.

Neo-Confucian philosophers began to regard Chi as emanating from the Great Ultimate (Tai Chi), the prime ordering principle of the universe. This school, whose ideas now predominate in traditional Chinese thought, held that Chi was transformed through the active yang and the passive yin modes into the Five Elements (Wu Hsing):

wood, fire, earth, metal, and water, which in turn formed the basic constituents of the physical universe.

They proposed that the human body, like matter in general, is made up of the Five Elements: wood, fire, earth, metal, and water. With these are associated other groups of five such as the five planets, the five conditions of the atmosphere, the five colors, and the five tones. Health, character, and the success of all political and private ventures were purported to be determined by the preponderance, at the time, of the yin or the yang, and the great aim of ancient Chinese medicine was to control their proportions in the body.

At the end of this period (circa 16th century), the monumental work *Pen Tsao Kang Mu*, *"The Great Pharmacopoeia,"* was written by Dr. Li Shizhen. This encyclopedic book comprehensively catalogued almost 2,000 herbs. This 52 volume work has been widely translated, frequently revised and reprinted, and is still used as an authoritative standard herbal today.

Confucius say, 'No way, Jose!'
With the adoption of Western medicine in modern China, one would expect the holistic, preventative practices of TCM to be found in the dumper. Could there be a place for gentle herbal medicine in a sea of surgery, antibiotics, and other powerful pharmaceuticals? Believe it or not, the answer is a resounding yes. I have been there and seen it with my own eyes. Because TCM is so engrained in Chinese culture, because it employs safe natural remedies, and because it so adeptly pinpoints the basic underlying causes of chronic disease, TCM has continued to thrive.

Under the scrutiny of today's modern science, the unsurpassable brilliance of TCM is actually asserting its clinical and pharmacological value. Western laboratories are beginning to dissect the mysteries of this ancient wisdom and actually validating it. In fact, progressive medical researchers are seriously trying to tap into it.

TCM works with the body's relationship with its individual parts and the environment. It also charges the individual with responsibility for his or her own health. According to TCM, health practitioners can only guide the individual through the healing process. Western medicine is based on the Cartesian philosophy, which views the body as a machine and only recognizes that which can be measured. In Western medicine, something is either mental or physical. In TCM, each organ has both a mental and a physical function.

In diagnosis, detailed questions are asked about the history of the illness and about such things as the patient's taste, smell, and dreams. Conclusions are drawn from the quality of the voice, and note is made of the color of the face and tongue. The most important part of the investigation, however, is the examination of the pulse. Based on work by Wang Shu-ho in the "Pulse Classic," written in the 3rd century BC, the pulse is examined in several places, at different times, and with varying degrees of pressure. This examination may take as long as three hours. It is often the only examination made, and it is used both for diagnosis and for prognosis.

Chinese herbs
In CHM, herbs are rarely taken singly. Rather, they are combined with several other synergistic herbs, sometimes upwards of 50 or more per formula. Prescriptions are tailored to the patient's specific needs. Five people with arthritis could each receive entirely different diagnoses and herbal treatments. Each formula will usually have a "chief" herb that goes after the main imbalance, an "assistant" to enhance the "chief," a "messenger" to guide to actions of the medicine to a particular body area, and a "harmonizer" that makes sure all the ingredients work together properly.

The demand for effective medicinal herbs is driving major advances in progressive modern medicine. Isn't it ironic that the traditions of Chinese medicine and the science of modern technology are starting to date? It's kind of like the complements of Yin and Yang coming together, contrary but co-dependent. My wife tells me opposites attract. That was us in 1987. Today we are one. Perhaps a paradigm that can contain the harmony of opposites holds the future to global health?

The herbs covered in this text that have strong foundations in Chinese medicine are: Aloe, Astragalus, Ginkgo, Scullcap, Dong Quai, Ginger, Ginseng, Horny Goat Weed, and Licorice.

Ayurvedic Medicine

Ayurveda is a 5,000 year old system of healing from India. The
word, Ayurveda, literally means the "Science of Life." Ayurveda is
based on the Vedas, the ancient Sanskrit texts that form the foundation of the Hindu religion. Since ancient times, the Vedas have
provided the primary philosophy and practice of traditional medicine
in India.

India's sacred teachings bled out beyond the Himalayas, most notably
to China. Hence, similarities are shared between Ayurveda and
Traditional Chinese Medicine, things like pulse diagnosis, the importance of keeping energy forces in balance, and the use of complex
herbal formulae used as therapeutics and preventatives. And, through
its impact on Mid-Eastern and Greek medicine, Ayurveda served as a
fountainhead from which Western medicine drank as well.

Under the British colonial rule of India, Western medicine became
official, and Ayurveda was temporarily disrupted. However, since
India's independence in 1948, Ayurvedic traditions have sprung back
into place, and now both forms of medicine coexist. In the U.S.,
Ayurveda shared a cup of coffee with Western medicine briefly in the
19th century but was soon abandoned as obsolete. One Ayurvedic
herbal medicine that enjoyed some popularity was Rauwolfia
serpentina, which yields reserpine, a cardiovascular drug that was
still around when I started in pharmacy in the 1960s.

Health is a feeling of well-being
Ayurveda defines health as a feeling of well-being; evenly balanced
emotional states; good memory and reasoning ability; properly
functioning senses; abundant energy; easy digestion; and healthy
functioning of bodily organs, tissues and other systems. Illness, on
the other hand, is thought to result from an imbalance, which must be
corrected by a combination of lifestyle changes and physical condi-
tioning including yoga, diet, and mental, spiritual and emotional
adjustments.

Ayurvedic healing practices are based on not only one's health, but
on one's individual constitutional type. There are three constitutional

types or *doshas*, and each of us is predominantly one type, though we each have elements of all three. They are *Vata* (air), *Pitta* (fire), and *Kapha* (earth).

Vata, Pitta, and Kapha

Vata types tend to be cold, slow digesters, who rarely perspire and fatigue easily. Those with a Vata constitution are creative, active, and quick learners. They adjust well to change but are worriers. Pitta types run hot, are hearty eaters, fast metabolizers, lean towards early graying or balding, are ambitious, and are good leaders. Kapha types tend to get heavy, are oily, move slowly, are tolerant, calm and loving, and are prone to envy.

The distinctions in determining constitutional types or doshas are far more complex than the few salient characteristics I am alluding to, and definitely beyond the scope of this book. The main point is that the herbs used in Ayurvedic medicine are matched not only to a person's health status, but also to his or her constitutional type.

The herbs included in this text which have their roots in Ayurvedic medicine are Guggul and Gymnema sylvestre.

Medicine of Ancient Egypt

The first physician to emerge is Imhotep, chief minister to King Djoser, in the 3rd millennium BC Carvings on the Karnak Temple, 1,500 BC, relate to botanicals, but it is the knowledge from the study of Ebers papyrus (1,700 BC), discovered in the 19th century, that gives us the most insight. The Ebers papyrus is a compendium of remedies, with appropriate spells or incantations, that lists the large variety of herbal medicines the Egyptians used. It mentions many common herbs like juniper and garlic. It also reveals some of the diseases suffered at that time including arthritis, tuberculosis of the bone, gout, tooth decay, bladder stones, and gallstones.There is evidence, too, of the parasitic disease schistosomiasis, which remains a scourge still.

Greek and Roman Influences

Hippocrates (460-370 BC)

Hippocrates is considered the father of Western medicine. He was the one to take medical thinking from superstition to science. He considered sickness to be a natural rather than supernatural phenomenon and believed that medicines should be administered civilly and without a magic ceremony. By the time Hippocrates practiced classical era Western medicine, it had taken in ideas from Western Asia and India. The philosophy of this time in the West was that diseases were the disturbances of the four humours, which were substituted for Yin and Yang. The four humours were black bile, yellow bile, blood and phlegm. Your health depended on their harmony at the moment.

Hippocrates invented clinical medicine. He practiced applications based on intelligent observations. He was a champion of patients' rights and the inventor of the bedside manner. He felt that it is the patient who matters, not medicine's theories of illness. He taught that the entire patient must be taken into account, including his or her surroundings. According to Hippocrates, "Ill health is a disharmony between man and his environment."

For his healing agents, Hippocrates used only all natural vegetables, fruits, seeds, and herbs. However, he wouldn't be considered an over-prescriber in that he believed, "Our natures are the physicians of our disease," which can be interpreted as, given a little help, the body is a self-correcting machine. Or, most people get well anyway.

Hippocrates invented holistic medicine 2,000 years before it was popular. He is regarded as a model for doctors and is said to have given medicine its soul. His most famous quote is, "Let your medicine be your food, and your food, your medicine." But he also said, "Do not judge the stool by its quantity, but by its quality." How can you not love this guy?

Theophrastus of Eresus (370-287 BC)
Theophrastus was a philosopher and friend of Aristotle. He is considered to be the Father of Botany. He wrote the first surviving herbal in 300 BC, called *Inquiry into Plants*. Under Theophrastus' organizational skills, the classification of plants blossomed into an ordered science.

he Elder (23-79 AD)

_ /as a Roman naturalist who was a prolific writer. His work, _The Natural History_, consisted of 37 books and was completed in 77 AD Books 12-19 cover botany and are his contribution to science. Although he is said to have drawn heavily on Theophrastus, he did contribute some independent observations, especially from his travels in Germany, and his text is a compilation of the beneficial herbs of his time.

Pliny was a pretty interesting character. He made it a point to live the good life. On a daily basis, he would take a cold bath, followed by a meal of raw foods. Then he would take siestas alternated between long writing sessions. His servant would read to him while he was in the bath and while he received his daily massages. He was eager to be an eyewitness of the eruption of Mt. Vesuvius. He strayed to close, and the rest is history.

Galen (131-200 AD)

Claudius Galen was born in Pergomon, in what is today Turkey. He was an avid collector of recorded knowledge and a prolific writer on medicine. He gained such a reputation in Rome that he was offered the post of physician to the Emperor Marcus Aurelius.

Galen established his own rules and classification of disease based on Hippocratic medicine. Even though he showed great respect for Hippocrates, when Galen was through, his highly complicated system was his own. In his diagnosis, he highly stressed the pulse. He believed in 'critical days' when men and women were more accident prone and gave diminished performance due, he believed, to the moon. Galen's system of healing essentially paralyzed European medical thinking for the next 1,400-1,500 years. Galenist physicians who followed him did not deviate from his system. When challenged, dogma always won out.

Galen left us something else. He was an overbearing man with an answer for everything. He set a personality pattern. He gave us arrogance in medicine.

Dioscorides (circa 129-210 AD)

For those of you with an eye for detail, Dioscorides, who supposedly lived from 129-210 AD, is also credited with having done something in 78 AD. Get over it. We are not really sure of any of these dates. He probably lied about his age for so long, track was lost.

Nevertheless, that doesn't make him a bad person. In fact, he was a great person. Dioscorides of Anazarbus is one of the great figures in the history of medicine and pharmacy. He was a Greek physician who accompanied Roman armies through their empire.

He left us the first illustrated textbook on drugs of all kinds called, *De Materia Medica*. There is no trace of famous Hippocratic-Galenic humoral pathology, although Dioscorides embraced Hippocrates from whose scrolls he pinched 150 descriptions of plants, which he added to his own work of over 600. Many of these plants are still used today and are easily recognizable from his primitive illustrations.

Galen quoted Dioscorides and gave him great respect for his work, while suspiciously ignoring Dioscorides' discussions on what the drugs did when administered to a patient for particular ailments. That would never have worked with Galen's tight proprietary systems. Nonetheless, Dioscorides' *De Materia Medica* remained a major work for over a thousand years.

Early Christianity Through the Dark Ages

In the words of Richard Gordon, in his incredibly entertaining book, *The Alarming History of Medicine:* "The early Christian Church resented doctors. They got in the way of the death business. The cause of disease was obviously sin; its treatment was prayer, fasting and repentance."

The Renaissance Influencer

Paracelsus (1493-1541)

Paracelsus was born Theophrastus Philippus Aureolus Bombastus von Hohenheim in the Swiss town of Ensiedeln. His father, a physician, chemist, and herbalist, was his first teacher. After his mother's death, Theophrastus traveled with his father through the Alps, while dad tutored him on medicine, herbs, minerals and metals. After settling in the little village of Villach, Theophrastus picked up his first life-changing piece of wisdom from Father Erhard, one of his teachers at a Benedictine monastery. He learned, "Knowledge gained through direct experience is primary."

With this pearl of wisdom under his 14-year-old belt, he set out to be a traveling student. He learned the practice of medicine from many sources, but he never really fit in. He was his own man, and he rejected Galen in exchange for the knowledge gained from his experiences. He became quite the rebel.

He used to begin his lectures by burning copies of Galen's books, rejected wearing the frocks prestigious doctors wore, and spoke in the German vernacular rather than Latin. He was very good at making people angry with him. He didn't care. He said the only person he was obligated to please was the sick patient he healed. Needless to say, Theoprastus spent most of his life traveling, staying one step ahead of the medical lynch mob.

By now, he had changed his name to Paracelsus. As a young medical student, he followed the teachings of the Roman physician Celsus, a disciple of Hippocrates. Celsus believed plant medicines should be used according to their activity, not their classification in the humoral system of healing. Very un-Galenic. He liked Celsus, but liked himself even more, so, never humble, he called himself, Para-Celsus, greater than Celsus.

By the end of his life, Paracelsus was to be remembered as a physician, chemist, alchemist, herbalist, metallurgist, and someone who always kept his bags packed. His accomplishments include: formalization of the Doctrine of Signatures (see below); the introduction into pharmacy of antimony, mercury and sulphur; the observation that sometimes the difference between a poison and a medicine is how much you give; moving medicine farther away from Galen; and teaching that diseases are specific entities and should be cured by specific remedies. Paracelsus could have been a product of the 1960s had he been born a few centuries later.

The Doctrine of Signatures

Before the availability of books and modern research techniques, the primitive populace had very little to work with when it came to predicting the medicinal effects of plants. They had trial and error, and appearance. If something worked, the information was passed on through generations to come.

A concept of "like curing like" seems to have developed independently in several parts of the world. It was used in China and India before 2,000 BC. The concept was based on the idea that plants, by their appearance, give clues to the medicinal virtues they may possess. Or, what a plant looks like, it cures. As mentioned above, the system was formalized by one of my favorites, Paracelsus, and became known as *The Doctrine of Signatures*.

For example, Paracelsus wrote the following about St. John's Wort: "The holes in the leaves mean that this herb helps all inner and outer orifices of the skin. The blooms rot in the form of blood, a sign that it is good for wounds and shall be used where flesh has to be treated." Today we know that this plant has been shown to be effective for mild to moderate depression, has anti-viral activity, and is an effective topical treatment for minor wounds.

Other examples of the Doctrine include: 1) Mandrake, with its tuberous roots for impotence. 2) Nutmeg, with its brain-shaped nuts for mental disorders. 3) White Willow and Quaking Aspen, with their fluttering leaves and branches for fever. 4) Eyebright, with its flower that resembles a pupil for eye problems. And of course 5) Ginkgo, with its bi-lobes resembling the brain for its cerebral circulation enhancement.

The Doctrine of Signatures influenced herbalism well into the 17th century, and still influences many African healers. This led to a fascinating study published in 1994. The author interviewed traditional healers in Zimbabwe about herbs they used to treat schistosomiasis, a urinary disorder characterized by blood in the urine. They produced three plants, Abrus prectorius, Pterocarpus angolensis, and Ozoroa insignis, all of which have either red seeds, red sap, or produce a red extract. The herbs were prepared in the typical manner and tested on laboratory animals infected with the parasite Schistosoma haematobium. All three herbs showed anti-schistosoma activity. Pterocarpus angolensis was even as active as the pharmaceutical praziquantel, and in addition, the plant had no side effects. Praziquantel, on the other hand, causes malaise, headache, dizziness, abdominal discomfort, rising temperature, and urticaria.

The 16th and 17th Centuries

John Gerard (1545-1611)

Gerard's contribution to medicine was his famous work, *The Herball, or Generall Historie of Plantes*, released in 1597. The *Herball* was immensely popular. It provided, in more than 800 chapters, information on species as they were then understood, common and botanical names, descriptions of habitats, time of flowering, and the "virtues," or uses of plants of the entire plant kingdom. It also contained a large amount of folklore. Substantial portions of the *Herball* were reprinted in 1927 and 1964.

Gerard was an Elizabethan physician, but if he were born today, with the freedom we now have to follow our dreams, he would have been a gardener. While studying medicine in London, he became interested in plants and began a garden near his cottage. He became herbalist to King James I, who also subsidized his garden. By the time the *Herball* was published, the garden, containing more than 1000 species, was as famous as Gerard was. And, a discussion of Gerard would not be complete if the fact that he was the first to grow potatoes in England weren't mentioned.

John Parkinson 1567-1650
Parkinson was the apothecary to Kings James I and Charles I, of England. His Herbal, *Theatre of Plants* (1640), containing 3,800 plants, is still, by many, considered the most comprehensive ever written in the English language.

Nicholas Culpepper 1611-1654
While destined to be a Cambridge trained doctor, young Culpeper fell in love and dropped out. Tragically, Culpepper's sweetie was struck by lightning and killed on their runaway rendezvous. A broken Culpepper still abandoned his studies but eventually became a pharma-

cist. He was drawn to the poor and became their "doc," like so many community pharmacists still are today, if there are any community pharmacies left.

Rather than prescribing expensive drugs, Culpepper would choose medicines people could get out of their own gardens. Paracelsus may have had this influence on him, as Paracelsus often advocated the use of local plants.

Culpepper knew that there weren't many pharmacists around with his medical school education. And, there were hundreds of thousands of people going without medical care because they couldn't afford it. So, he took it upon himself to raise the level of knowledge of his fellow pharmacists. He did this by translating the major medical works of the day from Latin into English.

This did not bode well with the "control freak" doctors of his day. Today's open-mined physicians would, of course, welcome anything that would bring better health care to more people. Culpepper was unfazed, having no use for these "proud, insulting, domineering doctors, whose wits were born five hundred years before themselves." The college of physicians countered with a smear campaign. They attacked his morals. They attacked his appearance, calling him "careless in his apparel," " a most despicable, ragged fellow."
Culpepper countered with a work that would make his name synonymous with the Herbal. His *English Physician* was a complete guide to health that allowed ordinary people to treat themselves with readily available, inexpensive remedies. It was an instant success and continued to be for centuries.

The Thomsonian Movement

Samuel Thomson (1769-1843) can be considered a medical reformer. The son of a poor farmer in New Hampshire whose health was frail, his childhood was bleak. Doctoring of the time had nothing to offer. His health made a drastic turnaround when his father called in a local herb doctor, the widow Benton. Young Samuel became fascinated by the use of plants and their healing powers.

A few regular doctors still prescribed herbs for their patients, but they were a dying class. The modern doctor was a breed of physician who relied on heroic efforts. They used toxic nostrums prepared from heavy metals like mercury, and then there was bleeding. The standard treatment for yellow fever was to bleed twice daily for ten days. Thomson felt "confident that the same treatment would kill half of those in health." The country was primed for change.

Thomson was a great observer and experimenter. He was especially drawn to the herbs lobelia and cayenne. Lobelia would cause vomiting by simply chewing the leaves. He theorized that this herb could act as a cleansing herb. The other herb that drew his fascination, cayenne, was a heating herb.

Thomson developed an entire philosophy of disease and a treatment plan for it. It was not very complicated. He believed that all diseases were caused by cold: "All diseases…are brought about by a decrease or derangement of the vital fluids by taking cold or the loss of animal warmth." Considering he lived in the northeastern United States, he may have been onto something. To cure disease, one must restore the vital energy and remove the obstructions the disease has generated. The obstructions, he said, were attached to the mucosal membranes of the stomach and bowels. Enter lobelia. To restore heat to the body, he would steam his patient and fire up their insides. Enter cayenne.

With this foundation, Thomson developed a series of treatments and patent medicines, using up to 65 different herbs borrowed from Native Americans. He was a great marketer. He was plain-spoken, obstinate, and a cantankerous crusader. His treatments enjoyed some success, probably due to a decrease in the death rate associated with treatment. Fame quickly sprang nationwide. By the late 1830s, Thomson claimed three million followers.

Thomsonianism did not do much for the relationship between the average American doctor and herbal medicine. Thomson's patented treatments had become almost as severe as the form of medicine he set out to change, and his success waned as other more sophisticated herbal approaches, better rooted in science came to be, namely the Eclectic movement.

The Eclectics

New Englander, Dr. Wooster Beach (1794-1868), like Samuel
Thomson, was not happy with the medicine of his day. He was drawn
to studying medicine, but, as he put it, "…my soul was filled with
indignation at these instruments of cruelty and misery, administered
under the specious pretext of removing disease." Burning with the
zeal of youth, he searched for an alternative.

He learned of an old German herbal doctor practicing in New Jersey,
with a successful practice, getting remarkable results. The more he
learned about Dr. Jacob Tidd, the more he wanted to know. He begged
Tidd to take him as a student, but he was turned down time after time.
As a result, Beach went into teaching and then business. For the next
seven years, he thought about medicine and continued to pester the old
Tidd. Impressed with the persistence of the young Beach, Dr. Tidd
finally gave in. Beach became his apprentice, and they worked side by
side over the next years.

After Tidd's death, Beach moved to New York and attended medical
school. He believed it was better to reform the system from within
than from the outside. He was also thinking ahead. The backlash to
Samuel Thomson's movement had brought about restrictive legislation
in many states, under pressure from medical societies. In New York,
for example, it was illegal to practice medicine without a diploma.
Having studied the Thomasonians in action, he wanted to make sure he
distanced himself from that movement. He felt Thomsonianism was a
total "subversion of all medical science" and based on the "ignorance,
prejudices and dogmas of a single individual."

Beach graduated school, was accepted into the New York Medical
Society, and began to practice. At first, he had hopped to win over his
colleagues. He felt by publishing in newspapers, periodicals, and
professional newsletters, the truth would prevail. Wrong. He was
branded a botanical outcast. He was backed into the same corner
Thomson had been years earlier: if the profession won't listen, go
directly to the customer. But, unlike Thomson, Beach was determined
to take on the profession on their own turf, with dignity, respect, and
along scientific lines.

He purchased some land in the City (New York) off of Grand, and, in 1827, put up a charming two-story building that he called "The United States Infirmary." From this Infirmary, he advertised a better system of medical and surgical practice. He enlisted young doctors who shared his ideas. In 1829, he erected another building alongside the first one, this time, a three-story structure, which was eventually named the "Reformed Medical College of the City of New York." Thus was launched the Eclectic movement.

The Eclectics became a group of North American physicians who selected from various medical disciplines what made sense. Their materia medica was almost entirely herbal based, much of which was borrowed from Native American medicine. They started their own medical journal called *The Western Medical Reformer*, and later, *The Eclectic Medical Journal* and *Ellingwood's Therapeutics*, some of which were published until 1920. Early Eclectic doctors were forced to make their own medicines, but by the 1840s, manufacturers were making ready-prepared drugs for them. One of these companies, H. M. Merrell and Co., was still in business during my early days in pharmacy in the early 60s. (Mind you, however, they were not manufacturing Eclectic herbal preparations anymore. They had shifted with the rest of the pharmaceutical mind-set.) The Eclectic movement also boasted several Eclectic medical schools around the country.

With the advance of orthodox science and the medical revolution with its brilliant advances in knowledge, herbal medicine, homeopathic medicine, and the gentle alternative natural approaches, were overshadowed. The straw that broke the Eclectic's back was the Flexner Report on Medical Education of 1910. This report established which medical schools were to receive public funding and which were not. This also had an effect on the direction philanthropic organizations, like the Andrew Carnegie coffers and the Rockefeller Foundation, would take. The result was all money going to orthodox medical schools. By 1920, seven of eight of the Eclectic schools were gone. By 1938, they were all gone. The monopoly enjoyed by the "old boy" medical community then still exists today.

Herbal Medicine in the 20th Century United States

Food and Drug Act of 1906

The history of herbal medicine in the 20th century United States is more a study of the law than of medicine. At the turn of the century, both the food and drug industry were in terrible condition. Abuses were more common than ethics. They included outrageous label claims, adulterations and substitutions, false labeling, deficient quality control, and even sanitation issues, although this was mostly a food problem.

The public became incensed and campaigned for laws to control food and drugs to better protect them. What resulted was often referred to as the Pure Food and Drug Act but was actually called The Food and Drug Act of 1906. It prohibited the sale of misbranded or adulterated drugs. Harvey Wiley, who was the man in charge of regulating food and drugs for the Department of Agriculture, was able to put an end to most of the worthless panacea medicines sold by charlatans from medicine show covered wagons. At the same time, keep in mind that the 1905 United States Pharmacopoeia also listed 191 legitimate plant medicines.

Food, Drug and Cosmetic Act of 1938

In 1937, the sulfonamide drug scandal set the public stage for the enactment of the Food, Drug and Cosmetic Act of 1938. Sulfanil-amide was the new antimicrobial drug of the day, and its manufacturer, Massengill Company wanted a dosage form that they thought might better appeal to the populace. It seems that in their mind, people from the South preferred to drink rather than swallow, so the Massengill Company embarked on a mission to develop an elixir of sulfonamide.

The problem came about when they selected diethyleneglycol as the agent to dissolve the poorly soluble drug. You see, diethyleneglycol is a close relative of the coolant we use in our car radiators. Over 100 people died from using the new elixir, and when the company was asked what kind of testing they performed before releasing the drug for sale, they admitted to only doing taste tests.

So, legislation was obviously necessary to ensure that the drugs being sold were safe. Hence, the Food Drug and Cosmetic Act of 1938 was passed. It required that all new drugs be proven safe before coming to market. All herbal medications were grandfathered in as they were assumed to be safe by virtue of their long history of use.

Kefauver-Harris Amendment of 1962

Things went along smoothly until thalidomide came along in the 60s. For those not old enough to remember thalidomide, it was an excellent anti-anxiety drug but, when prescribed to pregnant women, caused horrible birth defects. Senator Estes Kefauver from Tennessee, a friend of neither organized crime nor pharmaceutical companies (not that I am implying that there is a relationship), was so aroused by the tragedy that he carried legislation through Congress to further control the drug industry.

Kefauver was more successful with his bill than he was at running with Stevenson as a Vice Presidential candidate, and the Kefauver-Harris Amendment to the FDC Act of 1938 was passed in 1962. The amendment further defined what was considered safe and effective, and once again grandfathered the existing herbals.

The Food and Drug Administration, which incidentally was formed by the Food, Drug, and Cosmetic Act of 1938, was not at all happy with the herbal exemptions. They wanted to see botanicals controlled as drugs. So they did through regulation, what they couldn't do through legislation. They allowed the sale of herbs as usual, but regulated that no claims could be made for them unless those claims could be proven by the methods that were now required for drugs. If a claim were to be made, a manufacturer could bring supportive documentation before one of the FDA panels, but that documentation could not include anecdotal information from the medical community or patients, or the fact that the product worked and had done so for hundreds of years. The FDA wanted only sophisticated clinical trials that today would cost a manufacturer about $300 million dollars.

As you can imagine, not many claims were offered to the FDA for approval. Not even a pharmaceutical company would bring an herbal product to the FDA for approval because, after spending the necessary millions, a patent could not be secured to ensure a return on the investment since plants are in the public domain. Therefore, no patent protection and no market exclusivity would be granted.

Based on FDA regulations, only a handful of botanicals are considered legal drugs. Examples are Cayenne pepper cream for arthritis, Psyllium as a laxative, and Witch Hazel as an astringent. By FDA regulations, prune juice is not a laxative. So, in an effort to protect us, the government has over-protected us, and we have bureaucracy fighting science.

DSHEA

In 1993, the FDA, now under the direction of David Kessler, rattled its swords in the direction of removing herbs from the market as we know it, so as to have complete control of their use. Regulations were drafted and presented for public comment. Fortunately, the public commented. I understand that the only other issue that generated more mail to Congress was the Viet Nam war. As a result, Congress felt compelled to draft legislation to ensure that dietary supplements remained available to American citizens, and hence the Dietary Supplement and Health Education Act of 1994 (DSHEA) was passed. Under DSHEA, herbal products can continue to be sold without therapeutic claims. However, now the label can contain a structure and/or function claim. That means that you cannot say that a product kills infection, but you can say that it supports a healthy immune system. You cannot say that Hawthorn strengthens heart contractions or can lower blood pressure, but you can say that it supports a healthy cardiovascular system. And, if you choose to make a structure or function statement, you must print the following disclaimer, "This statement has not been evaluated by the Food and Drug Administration. This product is not intended to diagnose, treat, cure or prevent any disease."

Herbal Medicine in Europe

While we are arguing about prune juice in this country, most of Europe is light-years ahead of us. They allow therapeutic claims to be made for herbal medicines based on traditional use and reasonable certainty, with information coming from clinical and scientific literature, the medical field, the patients and folklore alike. In the case of Germany, in 1978, the government established a panel called Commission E to evaluate herbal health claims. They spent 15 years reviewing more than 300 age-old herbal remedies. Their efforts created a book of monographs, now published in English, which contains 191 approved herbs, 2 approved components, and 67 approved fixed combinations of herbs. *The Complete German Commission E Monographs* was a very valuable tool for my preparation of this book. German physicians prescribe herbs, and 12 percent of all German prescriptions are for herbal products. In fact, in Germany, the drugs of choice for depression, memory loss, and sinusitis are herbs.

Nomenclature

Man has been keeping lists of plants for as long as the ability to keep lists has been around. The Chinese have been doing it for 5,000 years, the Egyptians for 3,500 years, and the Assyrians for 2,700 years.

Theophrastus, in 300 BC, classified plants by their habitat or form (trees, shrubs, herbs), but also recognized sex characteristics between plants. This was a departure from previous approaches to classifying plants. Pliny the Elder followed with nearly a thousand plants in his Herbal, but these two works were pretty much copied and recopied until the sixteenth century, with little or no progress being made on plant classifications.

With the invention of printing, botany was elevated to the next level. Information could now be disseminated with ease, and the Age of Herbals was born. For the first time in 1,500 years, descriptive technique required herbalists to look at the plant rather than plagiarize the ancient Greeks and Romans. Plants now started to be grouped according to their morphological similarities rather than just their medicinal uses.

It didn't take long before a more sophisticated means of organizing plants was needed since about 4,000 kinds of plants were recognized at this point. Enter Carolus Linnaeus, 18th century botanist, whose influence is still felt in today's modern systems of classification.

In 1753, Linnaeus developed a system of classifying plants that included a hierarchy of formal rankings and a binomial naming system. He divided and subdivided based on the following categories: kingdom, division, class, order, family, genus, and species. The binomial system works just like our personal names work. Everybody gets a generic name based on the family they are in; mine would be Presser. And, then a specific name, to denote individual characteristics; so you can distinguish me from my sister, mine would be Art.

Linnaeus classified every plant known to him, all 7,300 species and 1098 genera. What he began is still used today; however, botanists consider the three most practical levels of classification to be the family, genus, and species.

Let's look at an example of Linnaeus' system, using peppermint.

Kingdom = plant

Division = Angiospermae, which means it is a flowering plant. This division contains over 250,000 specimens.

Class = Dicotyledoneae, which means the seeds have two lobes. This class contains 48 different orders and 289 families.

Order = Tubiflorae, which contains 26 families.
Family = Lamiaceae, which contains 200 genera and 3,000 species

Genus = Mentha, of which there are 25 different species.

Species = piperita, of which there is only one specimen.

The binomial name for peppermint is Mentha piperita L. The genus name is always capitalized, the species name is always lower case, and the L. at the end stands for the person who named the plant, in this case Linnaeus.

Plant Constituents

The politics of plant constituents

The therapeutic actions of plants have been known for sometimes thousands of years. Until modern science allowed us to, nobody really cared about what the chemicals were in the plants that were curing them. They cared only about the outcome. But, with the ability to identify chemicals, we are now in a better position to learn why the plant medicine is working.

However, plant chemistry has also played directly into the hands of the business of pharmaceuticals. No sooner did we start to identify the chemicals than we immediately tried to determine the active chemical. If it could be identified, it could be removed and used as a stronger and more predictable drug, although with greater toxicity.

For example, in 1785, Dr. William Withering (1741-1799), a "modern" physician of his day, was open-minded enough to follow up on a tip that the plant, foxglove, could be useful for what we would call today, congestive heart failure. The crude drug became digitalis. When we isolated the active chemical, a glycoside, it was removed, and the new drug became digoxin. With the patented medicine rave that has since come, digoxin is used much less than it used to be, having been replaced by monostructure unique chemicals that have a 17 year patent awarded to the manufacturer. Then, when a drug gets close to its patent date, the company comes out with a new and improved version, as with diazepam (Valium®), whose patent ran out allowing less expensive generics to be manufactured.

Deadly Nightshade (Atropa belladonna) yielded the alkaloid atropine. From the Poppy (Papaver somniferum) comes papaverine, and morphine. Pharmaceutical companies have not been interested in classics, but are, however, sending researchers into rain forests around the world looking for novel plants. Fifteen years ago, few or none of the top 250 pharmaceutical companies had plant research programs. Today, over half of them have such programs. The only problem is that less than 10% of the 250,000 known plants have been screened for their medicinal powers. And of those 250,000, some 60,000 species will probably become extinct by the year 2050. Somebody better hurry up and look for treasures.

Revival of interest originates from several areas, especially the fact that some companies are hitting home runs with being able to go right from plant, to active chemical, to changing the chemical into a synthetic analog, to testing, to market. Examples are the cancer drugs vincristine and vinblastine from Periwinkle, and the taxoids from the Pacific Yew tree. Historically, all drugs were derived from natural sources; currently, 25% of the drugs on the market have botanical origins.

Constituents

The major categories of plant constituents are proteins, carbohydrates, lipids, alkaloids, volatile oils, steroidal compounds, terpenoids, phenols, and glycosides. The chemistry of plants goes far beyond the scope of this book and could be a college course of its own. The highlights are as follows.

Proteins

This category is a gigantic group of macromolecules produced by plants. Twenty-two amino acids can be hydrolyzed from plant protein, just like animal protein. The plant uses amino acids and groups of amino acids, which we call polypeptides, to carry out specific cellular functions, both internally and externally. Plant proteins are also storehouses of nitrogen and protect the plant against would be predators.

Drugs have been developed from the amino acids derived from plants. L-Dopa, from fava beans, is used in the treatment of Parkinson's disease. L-Cysteine, found in all plants, is used in eye drops and topical antibiotics.

Proteins make up enzyme systems. Polypeptides can bend around and contort themselves, creating a unique receptor site for a particular chemical reaction to fit into, like a key into a lock. Proteins can combine with carbohydrates forming glycoproteins. Glycoproteins are many times associated with the immune system. Chlorophyll is a complicated protein derivative. It is actually called a porphyrin, which, in the case of chlorophyll, is a complex nitrogenous ring wrapped around a copper atom.

Carbohydrates
Carbohydrates are the fuel depot for plant energy. They are made up of sugar units. Monosaccharides and disaccharides are made up of one and two sugar subgroups and include glucose, fructose, sucrose, lactose, etc. Polysaccharides are made up of many sugar subgroups and include starches, inulin, etc. Through cellular chemical reactions, including respiration, other chemicals are produced from plant carbohydrates including acids, alcohols (like sorbitol and cellulose), and mucilage subgroups.

Plant carbohydrates have been a source of many useful pharmaceutical agents, but for the purposes of botanical medicine, polysaccharides and mucilages are of primary concern. Polysaccharides are known to exert beneficial effects on the immune system.

Mucilage is made up of polysaccharides that have the ability to soak up water forming a sticky gel-like mass. When consumed, this mass lines mucosal membranes reducing throat, lung, kidney and urinary irritation. Probably the most pronounced effects of mucilage lie in its ability to line the GI tract, reducing bowel irritation, acidity, and inflammation.

Lipids
Plant oils, unlike animal oils, are unsaturated fats. These are the oils you would purchase in the market, namely, olive, peanut, safflower, soybean, sunflower, corn, sesame, and canola oils. With the exception of olive oil, all these oils are extracted from plant seeds, the greatest source of plant oils. Plant oils can also be expressed and purified for use as supplements. Examples would include, primrose oil, flaxseed oil, and jojoba oil.

Two other subcategories within the lipids are waxes and phospholipids. Waxes are generally solid at room temperature and provide the durable, protective covering for plant leaves and fruit coatings. These waxes have been harvested for use in producing beeswax, carnauba wax (from leaves of Brazilian wax palm), and candelilla wax (from the coating on candelilla shrubs.)

Phospholipids are found in the cell membranes of plants. Chemically, they are a double lipid layer sandwiched between two layers of protein. Their value to the plant lies in their ability to act as an interface between fat-soluble and water-soluble materials. The most familiar phospholipid to the natural supplement industry would be lecithin from soybeans.

Alkaloids
Alkaloids are derived from amino acids and represent a very mixed group of nitrogen bearing, pharmacologically active molecules. They are, without doubt, the most therapeutic chemicals derived from plants and the category from which most pharmaceutical drugs have been manufactured.

Some examples of well known alkaloid-derived drugs are:

> ➢ Vincristine, derived from Madagascar periwinkle, used to treat cancer

> ➢ Atropine, found in deadly nightshade, used to reduce spasms, relieve pains and dry up bodily secretions

> ➢ Papaverine and morphine from the poppy, used to relieve pain.

> ➢ Reserpine, from snakeroot, an old blood pressure drug
> ➢ Colchicine, from autumn crocus, for gout

> ➢ Nicotine, from tobacco, a mild central nervous and strong cardiovascular stimulant

> ➢ Ephedrine, from Chinese ephedra (ma-huang), used for the relief of allergy symptoms and as a stimulant

> ➢ Quinine, from the bark of the cinchona tree, used in the treatment of malaria
> ➢ Capsaicin, from chili peppers, for pain relief

> ➢ Cocaine, from the coca shrub, for pain relief

> ➤ Caffeine, from the coffee bean, used as a stimulant and
> diuretic

and... the list could go on forever. All of these are alkaloid drugs.

Alkaloids are sensitive to heat, crystalline in structure, bitter, odorless, and alkaline in nature. More than 100,000 different alkaloids have been discovered in species from over 300 plant families, and new ones are being discovered at a rapid pace. Alkaloids have a pronounced effect on the human nervous system, but depending on the subgroup of chemical structure they fall into, be it indole, indolizidine, steroidal, purine, pyrolidine, tropane, solanaceous, pyridine, piperidine, muscarine, amine, capsaicin, quinolizidine, or a quinoline alkaloid, their activity is extremely diversified.

Some of the actions of alkaloids on the body include: antispasmodic, central nervous system stimulant, vasodilitation, bronchodilitation, diuretic, diaphoretic, analgesic, sedative, cytostatic, antileukemic, antimalarial, anti-arrhythmic, antibacterial, antiprotazoal, anesthetic, and this list could be endless.

Volatile oils
Volatile oils are responsible for the odor of plants. They contain hundreds of constituents, but the most common are terpenes, phenolic compounds that contain a six-carbon benzene ring, giving them their aromatic quality. For the plant, volatile oils serve several functions including repelling fungi and harmful insects, and providing the sweet fragrances of flowers that attract insects for pollinization.
Therapeutically, volatile oils have varied uses. Topically, they are used as antiseptics, tissue stimulants, and vasodilators. Internally, they can stimulate secretions, and have antibacterial, antispasmodic, sedative, expectorant, and antiseptic properties, in addition to being anti-inflammatory. Tea tree, for example, is known to contain a myriad of volatile compounds, many of them being strongly antiseptic. German chamomile contains a volatile oil that contains sesquiterpenes, such as azulenes, which have an anti-inflammatory effect.

Steroidal compounds

Technically, a steroid is a compound that contains four specifically arranged carbon rings, three six-sided, and one five-sided. From that point, steroids are differentiated by the side chains attached to the nucleus. If a sugar is attached to the steroid nucleus, a glycoside is formed. Steroid compounds are present in both animals and plants. They make up sex, anti-inflammatory, anabolic, and stress hormones, and are the basis for vitamin D, and bile salts and cholesterol. And, in the case of glycosides, steroids provide the precursors of a class of cardiac actives.

In plants, steroidal compounds are generally divided into steroidal alkaloids and saponins, with saponins being further divided into terpenoid saponins and steroid saponins. Saponins get their name from their characteristic lathering, like soap, when agitated under water.

Many plants containing steroidal saponins have marked hormonal activity, licorice, being one of the best known. Other saponins are often strong expectorants, anti-inflammatory agents, adaptogenic, anti-lipidemic, anticancer, antiseptic, immuno-stimulatory, and antioxidant agents.

Terpenoids

Terpenoids are the largest group of plant compounds. They are technically defined as natural compounds whose structure may be divided into isoprene units, a five-carbon branched chain molecule, also called isoprenoids. This class of plant compound is also referred to as terpenes.

Terpenoids are further subdivided into monoterpenoids, sesquiterpenoids, diterpenoids, triterpenoids, tetraterpenoids, caro-tenoids, and terpene lactones. Terpenoids are mentioned often in this text for their wide variety of medicinal actions. They activate the body's protective enzymes, protect the eyes, act as antioxidants, modify hormones, help block cholesterol absorption, reduce platelet aggregation, modify autoimmune conditions, balance nervous system disorders, protect cellular differentiation, stimulate gastric and mu-cosal secretions, and are antimicrobial, anti-inflammatory, anticancer, and adaptogenic.

Some terpenoids are unique to one plant. This is the case of Ginkgo biloba. Ginkgo contains diterpenoids called ginkgolides indigenous only to this one plant. Ginkgolides, as present in Ginkgo, are now used for a multitude of health challenges including memory loss.

Phenols

Phenols, or phenolic compounds, are widely distributed throughout the plant kingdom. They are chemically characterized by having an aromatic ring with one or more hydroxyl groups hanging on it. This parent group contains many subgroups referred to over and over again in this text. Those subgroups are polyphenols, anthocyanidins, catechins, flavonoids, and tannins. From the perspective of the plant, these phenols are intimately involved in the protection and survival of the species.

Flavonoids constitute about one-half of the 8,000 or so recognized phenols. Their medicinal actions, which overlap with the actions of many of the other members of this category, include being antioxidants, stress modifiers, anti-allergic agents, antiviral compounds, anticarcinogens, protein synthesis stimulators, anti-inflammatory, antispasmodic, antimicrobial, and vaso-protective agents. Isoflavones have strong antioxidant action in addition to helping balance hormones.

Anthocyanidins are a group of flavonoids, the pigments that give flowers and fruits a blue, purple, or red hue. Blackberries and grapes, as well as bilberry, contain appreciable quantities of anthocyanidins with a wealth of health benefits, many of which revolve around blood vessel integrity.

Tannins are produced to a greater or lesser degree in all plants. The harsh, astringent taste of tannin-laden bark and leaves makes them unpalatable to insects and grazing animals. Tannins contract tissues, hence their use to tan leather. Tannins are astringent; they draw the tissues closer together and improve their resistance to infection. They are also useful for the treatment of burns and to arrest bleeding. Additionally, tannin-containing plants have been used to treat diarrhea and nasal congestion.

Polyphenols in grape skins and seeds have been shown to inhibit plaque build up in arteries, increase HDLs that carry cholesterol away from the arteries, reduce blood clotting, act as antioxidants, and prevent mutations and tumor formation. And, if you think that is impressive, wait until you read about what catechins in green tea can do. Perhaps the two best beverages to consume are green tea and wine. Sounds good to me.

Glycosides

Glycosides are complicated compounds that breakdown into one or more sugars, called glycones, and a non-sugar component, called an aglycone. Glycosides are not a major component of plants, as are alkaloids, terpenes, or phenols. However, it is when one of these components combines with a sugar forming a glycoside that many of them take on a specific therapeutic action.

For example, when anthracenes combine with sugars to form anthraquinones, they take on their characteristic laxative effects. These are the actives in senna, aloe, and cascara. When the triterpenoid alkaloids in foxglove combine with sugars, they form the cardiac glycosides that have a strong, direct action on the heart, helping to support its strength and rate of contraction when it is failing. And, when coumarin becomes a coumarin glycoside, it takes on its medicinal effects, which are hemorrhagic, anti-fungicidal, and anti-tumor activities.

Plant Classifications used by Herbalists

Traditional herbalists classify herbs into five major categories based on their active constituents. These descriptions are a little variation on the discussion of plant components discussed above. The five categories are:

> ➤ Aromatic (volatile oils)
> ➤ Astringent (tannins)
> ➤ Bitter (phenolic compounds, saponins and alkaloids)
> ➤ Mucilaginous (polysaccharides)
> ➤ Nutritive (food stuffs).

Aromatic herbs

Aromatics owe their properties mainly to volatile oils. The name, "aromatic," is a reflection of the pleasant odor of many of these herbs. Volatile oils vary widely chemically, but most often are phenolic in nature (e.g., menthol from peppermint). The aromatic herbs are divided into two subcategories, stimulant herbs and nervine herbs.

Stimulant herbs most often affect the respiratory, digestive and circulatory systems. Examples include cayenne, garlic, ginger and feverfew. Nervine herbs affect not only the respiratory, digestive, and circulatory systems, but also the nervous system. Examples include chamomile, dong quai, hops and valerian.

Astringent herbs

Astringents owe their properties mainly to their tannins. Systemically, tannins have the ability to precipitate proteins, which "tightens" or tones living tissue. They usually affect the digestive, urinary and circulatory systems. On an ongoing basis, however, large doses of some astringents may sometimes be toxic to the liver. Examples of astringent herbs include comfrey, goldenseal, pau d'arco, white willow, and black walnut.

Bitter herbs

Bitters owe their properties to the presence of phenols and phenolic glycosides, alkaloids or saponins. They may be further divided into four subcategories: laxative herbs, diuretic herbs, saponin-containing herbs, and alkaloid-containing herbs.

Laxative herbs come in three basic types: bulk laxatives (mucilaginous herbs), lubricant laxatives (mineral oil), and stimulant laxatives (bitters). Stimulant laxatives are the kind that cause contractions and contain phenolic derivatives called anthraquinones. Examples are cascara, senna, aloe (outer leaf), and yellow dock.

Diuretic herbs induce loss of fluid from the body through the urinary tract. The fluids released through the urine eliminate toxins and excess liquid. Examples include buchu, dandelion, hawthorn, juniper berries, parsley and uva ursi.

Saponin-containing herbs have detergent properties that can result in the emulsification of fat-soluble molecules in the digestive tract. Saponins' most important property is to accelerate the body's ability to absorb other active molecules. Some saponins are also diuretic and antispasmodic. Examples include wild yam root, schizandra, licorice, black cohosh, yucca, ginseng and gotu kola.

Alkaloid-containing herbs are some of the most potent drugs known today. The general definition of an alkaloid makes an herb classification difficult since each group of alkaloids has very different physiological effects. Many alkaloid-containing herbs are also found under additional classifications (e.g., valerian and cayenne). Examples of alkaloid-containing herbs include ephedra, goldenseal, valerian and cayenne.

Mucilaginous herbs
Mucilaginous herbs derive their properties from the polysaccharides they contain. Most mucilages are not broken down by the human digestive system but absorb toxins from the bowel and give bulk to the stool. The major effects of mucilaginous herbs are to speed up bowel transit time, absorb toxins, and regulate intestinal flora. Mucilaginous herbs are demulcent (soothing) and vulnerary (wound healing). Examples include aloe vera (gel from inner fillet), comfrey, psyllium, and slippery elm.

Nutritive herbs
Nutritives owe their name and classification to the nutritive value they provide to the diet. They are foods that exert some mild medicinal effects such as providing fiber, mucilage and diuretic action. Most importantly, they provide macronutrients and/or micronutrients. Examples include rosehips, barley grass, bee pollen, spirulina and wheat germ.

Dosage Forms

A variety of commercial dosage forms are available in the marketplace today. They stretch from the simplest holistic preparations on one end of the spectrum, to the most purified pharmaceuticals on the other end.

Whole plant

Using the whole plant, as the Maker provided it, is the most basic herbal preparation. We often call this "whole plant," but we mean that we are using the appropriate part of the plant (root, leaf, flower) in its entirety. That is, we are drying it, grinding it into a powder, and encapsulating it. The advantage to using whole plant capsules is that you get everything that is in the plant, just as it grew. The disadvantage is that often the potency might be too low to be a good medicine.

The way to get more bang for the plant buck is to take the chemicals out of the plant and concentrate them. This is what you are doing when you use an extract.

Tea

When you steep a tea bag, you are making an extract called an infusion. If you cook herbs, you are making an extract called a decoction. Either way you end up with plant chemicals in water. The disadvantage to teas is that you are only able to extract the components of the plant that are soluble in water. This is fine if you are only interested in plant components like polysaccharides, but if not, you miss many of the other beneficial plant compounds.

Having said that, let me make a 180 degree turn and state that Traditional Chinese Medicine (TCM), the oldest herbal medicine, is based on teas. TCM is a teapot medicine. Herbs are gathered and cooked all together. I have done this. It's not very pretty, and it doesn't taste very good. But you can't argue with success.

Tinctures

A tincture is an extract of an herb in a mixture of alcohol and water. Plant material is chopped and allowed to soak in the hydroalcoholic mixture for a couple of days. When the plant material is separated from the liquid, it contains a given amount of soluble plant mass.

When preparing an extract using alcohol and water, many choices must be made. The more alcohol you use, the more of the lipid-soluble compounds you will extract. The more water you use, the more water-soluble compounds you will extract. You can choose to perform a full spectrum extraction or you can choose to extract for a single active component or family of components. This is all done by manipulating the solvents.

For a full spectrum extract, you choose the amount of alcohol and water that will bring out the maximum of plant matter. If you started with 100 gm. of plant material and were able to recover 25 gm. of plant solids at the end, you have created a 4:1 extract.

To prepare an extract targeting an active or a marker chemical, the solvents are manipulated to capture the solubility of the chemical you are going after. These kinds of extracts are referred to as standardized extracts.

Fluid extracts

Fluid extracts are similar to tinctures except that during the extraction process, solvent is distilled off to concentrate the extract. The end result is 1 gm. of plant solids in 1 gm of solvent.

Solid extract

A solid extract is a fluid extract from which all the solvent has been removed. This is the product used in tablets and capsules and is generally considered the most concentrated herb form.

The great herbal controversy

Which is best, whole herb, full spectrum extracts, or standardized extracts? The answer is not cut and dry, but a statement of facts. The further you get from the way the plant was made by the Maker, the more complications and side effects you will introduce into the equation. Nature knows what she is doing when she puts hundreds of chemicals into a plant all working in synergy. So, based on that fact, a full spectrum extract would be closer in touch with Nature.

However, you cannot turn your back on science. If 200 studies are done with a particular standardized extract with positive outcomes, how could you want to use anything else? When clinical studies are conducted, and they determine that the effectiveness of their results was based on delivering a given number of milligrams of what is believed to be an active compound, why argue with success?

So, when all is said and done, go with the science. Do what has been proven clinically.

Cautions

"Not everything that can be counted counts, and not everything that counts can be counted"— *Albert Einstein*

The new generation of skull and bone reporters

Herbs are generally extremely safe with little if any toxicity or even side effects associated with them. However, I can't help but notice that herb bashing has become very popular. It is politically correct for mainstream medicine cronies to declare herbs as uncontrolled, unsafe, and having no place in healthcare. Mainstream medicine is a "good ole boys" club, and they don't like change. They would like us to think that all herbs will either interfere with prescribed medication, or adversely affect the disease pathology being treated, or create a third problem. That works better for them and the pharmaceutical companies, although many pharmaceutical houses are hedging their bets and getting into the herb business.

So many publications have appeared on the market of late, each with long lists of herb-drug interactions and serious contraindications. Where did these come from? Being one of the first mainstream pharmacists to jump to the natural side over twenty years ago, shouldn't I have come across some of these problems? I have never seen a significant problem someone has gotten him or herself into by taking herbs. How come the Europeans, who are light-years ahead of us in integrating herbs into their mainstream medical system, haven't come across all these potential problems?

I solved the mystery. After closer scrutiny, I find the words "speculative," "theoretical," "empirical," "a rat study," "a letter to the editor." And where does the theory and speculation come from? From studies done with the plants? No. It is coming from pharmaceutical mentality. And what is pharmaceutical mentality? It is mono-structure single entity chemistry. That is what drugs are. A single chemical. A single, unnatural chemical. A new drug is a single chemical never formulated before. Then comes the patent. Then comes the price gouging.

A drug is its parts (parts equaling one). A plant is not its individual parts. A plant can have hundreds of significant chemicals identified in it. But it is not any of those chemicals. A plant is the sum of its parts and must be evaluated as a whole. Every time you take a step away from Nature, you run the risk of side effects and complications. When you pull one chemical out of a plant, you are no longer are talking about the plant, you are talking about a drug. Even extracts that are highly standardized to one phytochemical still have all the other constituents remaining in the extract. They are not just a single chemical.

The way the new breed of herbal safety evangelists are generating potential interactions and contraindications is to look at the individual chemicals in a plant and "speculate" that because that chemical may be a problem, the whole herb could be a problem. Providing extensive lists of "theoretical" side effects and toxicities has become the new fashionable way to sell books, especially those targeted to conventional health professionals. In most cases, the "theorized" toxicity or potential untoward effect has nothing to do with the way the *Maker* provided the botanical, that is, in its totality of components.

When Mother Nature manufactures a product, she knows what she is doing. If she accidentally put a poison in her plant, she probably included the antidote. If she put in a blood-thinning chemical into the mix, and she didn't intend this plant to be used for this purpose, she probably put a coagulating agent into her recipe. If she put a cancer-causing chemical in her plant, she added a cancer drug to the soup. If she put a chemical in her plant that raises blood sugar, she probably put it in to enhance glucose utilization. She knows her business. An herb is not its parts. It is the sum of its parts and should be evaluated that way.

Watch out for Alfalfa

It didn't take me long to come across these new tactics. I started this book with Alfalfa. One source warns that because of its coumarins (blood thinning phytochemicals), alfalfa should not be used by people taking blood-thinning drugs because it could over thin their blood. O.K. Another source says, "Excessive use of herbs that contain vitamin K, an essential coagulation factor, can increase the risk of clotting in people using anticoagulants. These herbs include

Alfalfa, Parsley, Nettle, Plantain, and others." Come on, guys. The least you can do is read each other's books. The truth is that the *Maker* built his car to be driven. He covered his bases. The effect is a wash—especially since this whole exercise is theoretical.

Green tea and clotting

Here is another example of what you get when you look chemical by chemical. Following are the opinions of two sources: "Consumption of large amounts of green tea provide a significant source of vitamin K that can antagonize the effect of warfarin." "Green Tea can prolong bleeding time and increase the results of a bleeding time test." Make up your mind guys. By the way, opinion number two is correct.

Ginger is poison

Ginger is another good example. Ginger is a food substance and spice that has been ingested every day, in significant amounts, by millions of people throughout the history of the world. It is an extremely safe substance. In fact, if you were to search the medical literature for cases of ginger toxicity or untoward effects, whether used as a food or a medicine, you would be hard pressed to turn something up.

Ginger is so safe that I could not find an LD_{50} on this herb. An LD_{50} is a test of toxicity. It stands for lethal death 50%, which I always found a curious phrase (can you have a non-lethal death?). It is the amount of a substance, expressed in mg per kg of body weight, necessary to produce death in 50% of the population tested (a good job not to volunteer for). An LD_{50} could not be established for Ginger, not because they couldn't find volunteers; laboratory animals are used, and they do not get to vote. It could not be established because it is impossible to feed a rodent enough Ginger to kill it.

The pungent chemicals that give Ginger its primary medicinal qualities are called 6-gingerol and 6-shogaol, and they do have an LD_{50}. When these chemicals in Ginger were tested, it was determined that one would have to consume up to 9,000 times the normal dose of Ginger to have a 50-50 chance of a fatal outcome. When you extrapolate that to dried powdered Ginger, as you would take in a capsule, you would have to consume about 20 pounds.

In 1982, the safety of Ginger was questioned when the media reported that Ginger could be mutagenic. This newsflash was based on a study that concluded that an isolated chemical in Ginger can accelerate mutagenicity of mutagenic chemicals in a plate full of bacteria in a laboratory. However, the study was flawed in that no activating or inhibiting enzyme systems were used, as required by the standard test for mutagenicity. Ooops!

Additionally, the researchers found that Ginger contains powerful antimutagneic chemicals that prevent mutagenicity. Ginger also contains powerful antioxidants that should have been considered. In fact, when all was said and done, the researchers concluded that whole Ginger was probably not mutagenic. The truth be known, Ginger actually has been shown to prevent mutagenesis by the standard mutagen, tryptophan pyrolysate.

Another example, using Ginger while we are on the subject, is the warnings in the alarmist publications against its use with anticoagulant and antiplatelet drugs. A book states, "Theoretically, excessive amounts might increase the effect or the risk of bleeding." Here again we have speculation, and how much is *excessive*?

When reviewing the literature, we find that investigators have examined Ginger for its blood thinning effects because one of its components has aspirin-like pharmacology. So, they tested Ginger for its blood thinning properties. What they found was that 4 grams daily of powdered Ginger (the equivalent of 8 capsules of 500mg each), for three months, did not alter various measurements of blood coagulation in humans. At a single dose of 10 grams (the equivalent of 20 capsules of 500mg each), reduced platelet aggregation was discovered. However, another trial concluded that 15 gram daily doses, probably divided (the equivalent of 30 capsules of 500mg each), for two weeks, had no anti-thrombotic effect in humans. So, I once again have to ask, "How much is *excessive*, and should the general public be warned not to take 20 capsules of Ginger at once if they are taking blood thinning drugs?"

Bless the media

The media understands herb bashing. They are the specialists in
negative news. How about *Herbs Impair Fertility*, specifically
Echinacea and St. John's Wort. Here's the story. Researchers take
hamster eggs and strip them of their protective coating. They soak
them in the herbal extracts for an hour, then test to see if fertilization
will occur. No go.

How about the rest of the story. What if this were done in the human
body? First of all, the extract would have to be consumed and absorbed 100%, which is impossible. It would have to pass through the
liver unchanged, which it can't. The 100% fictitiously absorbed and
liver-immune extract would now have to find its way to an egg, all of
it. When it got there, it would have to sit there for an hour. Even if all
this is could happen, the concentration of the extract in the ovary is 1/6
the amount used in the study. Give me a break. Do you think the
public was misled?

Somebody handed me the Health section of the *New York Post*, dated
20 June, 2000, while I was on a business trip. He pointed to "Information that Can Save Your Life." It was an herb bashing article. The
warning he pointed to was don't mix Echinacea with drugs that cause
liver problems because Echinacea can cause liver problems. What?
Where does that come from? Well, maybe someone took the chemicals apart again. Echinacea has pyrrolizidine alkaloids, which have the
reputation of being hepatotoxic. This is the case in the herb Comfrey.
However, the rest of the story is that pyrrolizidine alkaloids with an
unsaturated nucleus are toxic. The ones in Echinacea are saturated, so
they are not toxic. Ooops! Take it back *New York Post*. Good luck.

The case of the hysterical anesthesiologist

In 1998, articles buzzed around the medical literature warning of the
danger of using St. John's Wort. This "danger-alert" was based on the
obsolete fact that St. John's Wort is an MAO inhibitor. MAO inhibitors should be discontinued two weeks prior to surgery. Well, I don't
know what effect St. John's Wort has on anesthesia, but we can safely
assure this California doctor that MAO inhibition has nothing to do
with its mechanism of action. I do, however, recommend discontinuing almost all herbs prior to surgery, especially anticoagulants.

Common sense

I think using herbs safely is mostly a little warning and mainly common sense. What I have tried to do is note problems that are more likely to be real and explain common sense options to dealing with them. I have a great deal of respect for pharmaceutical drugs and don't advocate discontinuing their use. Many times, options are available so that you can use both herbs and pharmaceutical drugs. Your physician is a part of your health team. So are you. You should be able to work together. If not, finding other physicians more in touch with today's options who are taking new patients shouldn't be difficult.

Pregnancy

When it comes to taking herbs during pregnancy, I come down on the side of no. Herbs are not warm fuzzies. They are natural drugs and should be treated that way. Unless I have specifically mentioned the use of an herb during pregnancy, or it has been screened by a body like the Commission E German authorities and rated as considered safe, don't do it.

Not all herbs are appropriate for children; however, in this text I have mentioned several that are. If the manufacturer of the product you purchase does not give a children's dose on the label, consider using one or both of the rules they taught us in Pharmacy school:
Clark's Rule: child's weight (in pounds) divided by 150 lbs, times the adult dose.
Young's Rule: child's age (in years) divided by (adult's) age (in years) plus 12, times the adult dose.

Conclusion

Herbs are not as scary as their detractors would lead you to believe. Drug therapy has been coming in at somewhere between the 4th and 6th leading cause of death. And that's for properly prescribed, properly administered drugs, too. That's right up there with heart disease and cancer. Perhaps those who rely on drugs should spend more time cleaning their own house before they start trying to scare you away from ours. Voltaire once said, "Doctors pour drugs of which they know little, to cure diseases of which they know less, into human beings of which they know nothing."

Botanical Medicine Today

Sixty million Americans use herbal medicines, or what conventional medicine is calling unconventional medicine. Billions of dollars are being spent on herbal medicines, probably fueled by my fellow baby boomers, who, as we age, are becoming more health aware and increasingly dissatisfied with conventional medicine's attempts to diminish the adverse effects of aging. And besides, my generation has always been dissatisfied with anything conventional.

It is estimated that 65% of people in the world use herbal medicine as their only line of medicine. According to the World Health Organization, the figure is 80%. How can it be called unconventional medicine? Perhaps the system of using mono-structure, single entity drugs should be called unconventional medicine?

Why have so many turned to herbals? I don't think there is one clear-cut answer but rather a series of answers. The United States is undergoing a movement towards self-care. People are beginning to take responsibility for their own health, and in a natural way. The population has taken an increased interest in wellness and has become aware of alternative approaches to healing.

To a certain extent, consumers have become disillusioned with the efficacy of conventional medical care. People are viewing the system as being significantly less than omnipotent based on its return on investment in diseases like AIDS, cancer and heart disease. With the money we have poured into these devastating diseases, people think we should be a little further ahead.

The American public is fed up with the lack of respect the medical system offers them. You have to wait in a lobby for an hour, only to be let into a holding room to wait another 15- 30 minutes, so you can spend the 6.5 minutes the HMO allows your doctor to spend with you, if you get a doctor and not a physician's assistant.
Herbal medicines are perceived as being gentle alternatives to pharmaceutical drugs. The public has become more concerned with the serious side effects of many modern drugs. They are getting smarter,

going on-line, learning more about the drugs they are taking, and not liking what they are finding out.

Many drugs have an addictive nature. Is there anybody reading this who hasn't had direct contact with someone who has had a problem with tranquilizers or pain pills? Prescriptions for these dangerous drugs are often given out like samples at a trade show.

The indiscriminate use of antibiotics has resulted in a crisis of resistant strains of organisms in this country. New microbes are emerging, and some of our old enemies are waging a comeback. Since 1929, when Sir Alexander Fleming discovered penicillin, we have been adding on new antibiotic on top of new antibiotic.

The overuse and misuse of antibiotics are the two greatest contributing factors to the desperate situation we find ourselves in today. Antibiotics are being inappropriately prescribed for the flu, a non-susceptible viral infection. Antibiotics are prescribed to just prevent infections, a practice designed to prevent secondary infections but only appropriate in a small, well-defined patient population. And, even when antibiotics are suitably prescribed, patients often are guilty of noncompliance, not taking their medication until it is all gone, as prescribed. The public is beginning to think they are better off using botanicals that can push our defenses in the direction of wellness.

More people are turning to botanicals just because of the sheer skyrocketing cost of drugs today. If you don't have insurance for your medicines, chances are you can't afford to use them. Even the costs of over-the-counter drugs have spiraled out of control. Herbs offer an inexpensive alternative.

The last two reasons the American public has turned to herbal medicines are that they are readily available, and they work. Herbs are not only readily available, they are, perhaps, too available. I am concerned that herbs are offered in outlets where consumers are not getting the level of care they should be getting when purchasing a medicine. I would be more comfortable if I knew that herbs were sold by competent and trained individuals.

As for the last reason the use of herbs has increased, the fact that they work, this is not news. Modern science is proving what the world has known for 5,000 years. Herbs work. If you are purchasing high quality herbs from reputable outlets, you are likely to get results based on science. However, not every herb will work for everybody; we don't even get those results with pharmaceuticals.

I am not advocating that everyone discontinue taking drugs and turn to herbs. I am a conventionally trained pharmacist and have the utmost respect for pharmaceuticals. They certainly have their place. What I do advocate is tolerance and open-mindedness. There are plenty of non-life threatening conditions where something non-toxic and natural can be tried before breaking out the heavy artillery. It is done every-where else in the world; it can be tried here.

References:

Beinfield, H, et al. "Chinese Traditional Medicine: An Introductory Overview." *Alternative Therapies*. 1995; 1:44-52

Beinfield, H, et al. *Between Heaven and Earth: A Guide to Chinese Medicine*. New York, NY. Ballantine Books. 1991

Bordia, A, et al. "Effect of Ginger and Fenugreek on Blood Lipids, Blood Sugar and Platelet Aggregation in Patients with Coronary Artery Disease." Prostaglandins Essent Fatty Acids. 1997; 56:379-84

Chin, W, et al. *An Illustrated Dictionary of Chinese Medicinal Herbs*. Sebastopol, CA. CRCS Publications. 1992

Dastur, J. *Everybody's Guide to Ayurvedic Medicine*. Bombay. D.B. Taraporevala Sons. 1960

Di Stefano, V. "Paracelsus: Light of Europe (Part 1-3)." *Australian Journal of Medical Herbalism*. 1994; 6: 1-3, pp. 5-8, pp. 33-36, pp. 57-60

Editorial, "Pharmaceuticals from Plants." *Lancet*. 1994; 343:1513-5

Griggs, B. *Green Pharmacy*. Rochester, VT. Healing Arts Press. 1991

Guh, J, et al. "Antiplatelet Effect of Gingerol Isolated from Zingiber Officinale." *J Pharm Pharmacol*. 1995; 47:329-32

Hoffmann, D. *The Information Sourcebook of Herbal Medicine*. Freedom, CA. The

Crossing Press. 1994

http://www.wam.umd.edu/-mct/plants/teach/pharmacognosy1html

Janssen, P, et al. "Consumption of Ginger Does Not Affect *In Vivo* Platelet Thromboxane Production in Humans." *Eur J Clin Nutr*. 1996 50:772-4

Jitoe, A, et al. "Antioxidant Activity of Tropical Ginger Extracts and Analysis of Contained Curcuminoids." *J Agric Food Chem*. 1992; 40:1337-40

Kada, T, et al. "Antimutagenic Action of Vegetable Factors on the Mutagenic Principle of Tryptophan Pyrolysate." *Mutation* Research. 1978; 53: 351-353

Kapoor, L. *CRC Handbook of Ayurvedic Medicinal Plants*. Boca Raton, FL. CRC Press. 1990

Lazarou J, et al. "Incidence of Adverse Drug Reactions in Hospitalized Patients." *JAMA* 1998; 279:1200-1205

McCaleb, R. "Possible Shortcomings of Fertility Study on Herbs." *HerbalGram*. 46; 22

Nagabhushan, M, et al. "Mutagenicity of Gingerol and Shogaol and Antimutagenicity of Zingerone in Salmonella/Microsome Assay." *Cancer Letter*. 1987; 36:221-3

Namakura, H, et al. "Mutagen and Antimutagen in Ginger, Zingiber Officinale." *Mutation Research*. 1982; 103:119-126

Nyazema, N. et al. "The Doctrine of Signatures or Similitudes: A Comparison of Efficacy of Prasziquantel and Traditional Herbal Remedies Used for the Treatment of Urinary Schistosomiasis in Zimbabwe." *Int J Pharmacog*. 1994; 32:142-8

Ondrizek, r, et al. "An Alternative Medicine Study of Herbal Effects on the Penetration of Zonafree Hamster Oocytes and the Integrity of Sperm Deoxyribonucleic Acid." *Fert Sterl*. 1999; 71:517-522

Robbers, J, et al. *Pharmacognosy and Pharmacobiotechnology*. Baltimore, MD. Williams & Wilkins. 1996

Southern Illinois University Carbondale/Ethnobotanical Leaflets/URL http://www.siu.edu/~ebl/ 1999

Stearn, W. *Botanical Latin*. Portland, OR. Timber Press. 1998

Sueckawa, M, et al. "Pharmacological Studies on Ginger. I. Pharmacological Actions of Pungent Constituents 6-Gingerol and 6-Shogaol." *J Pharm Dyn*. 1984; 7:836-48

Yamahara, J, et al. "Inhibition of Cytotoxic Drug Induced Vomiting in Suncus by a Ginger Constituent." *J Ethnopharmacol.* 1989; 27:353-5

Wilkinson, J. "The Signature of Plants." *Kindred Spirit.* 1997; 3:36-38

Part Two

Medicinal Herbs

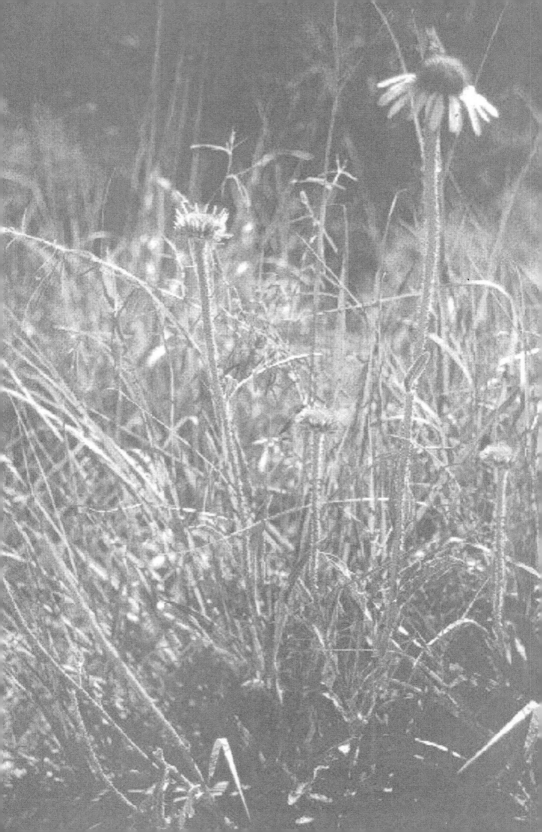

Alfalfa

(Medicago sativa)

Other Common Names:

Lucerne, Purple Medick, Medicago, Buffalo Herb

Background:

Alfalfa is mentioned in Chinese medicine dating back to 2939 BC The Arabs fed it to their horses, believed it improved the health and performance of their animals, and named the plant "al fal fa," the "father of all foods." Legend has it that the Greeks imported Alfalfa from the East, and Dioscorides, a 1st century physician, employed it to treat urinary disorders.

The medicinal uses of Alfalfa come from folklore and anecdotal reports. They include the treatment of kidney, bladder and prostate disorders, arthritis, digestive problems, diabetes, anemia, poor appetite, menstrual problems, breastfeeding problems, and high cholesterol.

Science:

Most herbal authorities consider Alfalfa more of a food than an herbal medicine. It is rich in protein and vitamins A, B-1, B-6, B-12, E, and K. Most studies that lead to possible benefits are done with animal models.

Alfalfa does contain a saponin fraction that is believed to offer cholesterol-lowering benefits. Animal studies do show that Alfalfa reduces cholesterol absorption by binding the fats.

Alfalfa contains plant enzymes that may assist in digestion. It also contains a substance referred to as Vitamin U, a nutrient also present in raw cabbage, which has been associated with the treatment of ulcers. This would be consistent with Chinese herbalist use of the herb to treat ulcers.

Modern Day Uses:

In my opinion, for whatever Alfalfa has been claimed to do, better studied and more clinically sound herbs exist. However, I have talked to people who swear by it. If someone wanted to use Alfalfa as an alkalinizing agent to treat ulcer conditions, arthritis, or to increase breast milk production, I would not strongly resist. Also, if someone were seeking a vegetarian nutritional supplement and wanted to include Alfalfa as part of their regimen, I would encourage him.

Dose:

Since Alfalfa is more of a food than a medicine, use it aggressively. I generally recommend 9-18 tablets daily in divided doses.

Cautions:

Reports of toxicity relate only to the seeds and sprouts of Alfalfa and not the dried leaves used in supplements. A relationship may, however, exist between large doses and the long term use of Alfalfa, and an exacerbation of the symptoms Systemic Lupus, an autoimmune disease. It has to do with l- canavanine, an amino acid in Alfalfa that is an analog of arginine.

References:

See General Resources

DerMarderosian, A ed. *Review of Natural Products*. St. Louis, MO, Facts and Comparisons, 1999

Duke, J. *The Green Pharmacy*. Emmaus, PA, Rodale Press. 1997

Lust, J. *The Herb Book*. New York, NY. Bantam Books. 1983

Mowrey, D. *Herbal Tonic Therapies*. New Canaan, CT. Keats Publishing. 1993

Roberts, J, et al. "Exacerbation of SLE Associated with Alfalfa Ingestion." *New Eng J Med*. 1983; 308:1361

Santillo, H. *Natural Healing with Herbs*. Prescott, AZ. Hohm Press. 1993

Tierra, M. *The Way of Herbs*. New York. Pocket Books. 1990

Aloe

(Aloe barbadensis, A. spp.)

Other Common Names:

Aloe Vera, Cape Aloe, Zanzibar Aloe, Socotrine Aloe, Curacao Aloe, Barbados Aloe, Burn Plant, Elephant's Gall, First-Aid Plant, Hsiang-Dan, Lilly of the Desert, Lu-Hui, Medicine Plant, Miracle Plant, Plant of Immortality, Venezuela Aloe

Background:

Aloe Vera is a succulent member of the lily family, originating in Africa, where most of the genus Aloe are indigenous. The name Aloe is from the Arabic *alloeh*, or Hebrew *halal*, meaning a shining bitter substance. The inner leaf contains a slimy gel used in medicines and cosmetics. The outer leaf tissue contains the yellow bitter juice which is known as aloe drug or "bitter aloe," and is used primarily as a laxative. Today, Aloe is commercially grown in the Southwest and Mexico.

King Solomon, Cleopatra, Marco Polo, and zits?

Historical and religious documents of the Egyptians, Romans, Greeks, Hebrews, Chinese, and more, make reference to this healing plant over a span of 4,000 years. Aloe was included in a list of herbs and plants that grew in King Solomon's gardens. An ancient Egyptian papyrus mentions Aloe 12 times in various preparations. According to legend, Nefertiti and Cleopatra used it to enhance their beauty, and Alexander the Great conquered Socotra because he wanted the Indian Ocean island for its famed Aloe supplies, which he wanted to heal his troops' wounds.

Marco Polo reported that the Chinese used Aloe to allay, among other ailments, gastric distress and rashes. The great 1st century Greek healer Dioscorides, who accompanied Roman armies as a physician, used Aloe for wounds, stomach pain, digestive disorders, constipation, headache, itching, baldness, mouth and gum diseases, kidney ailments, blistering, sunburn, and blemishes. Who would have thought that *zits* were an issue in the 1st century?

Columbus' ship log refers to medicinal uses of Aloe for his sailors. Spanish missionaries brought Aloe with them to America. However, it wasn't until the 1930s that Aloe saw modern clinical use with its successful treatment of burns caused by primitive X-ray and raduim treatments.

However, mainstream medicine still tends to turn its nose up to Aloe and will probably continue to relegate the plant to "folk remedy" status, at least until its mechanisms of action become less elusive. Like most botanicals, a lack of financial incentive discourages the investment of the necessary millions of dollars necessary for research. Most work on Aloe is undertaken by university researchers with limited budgets, often in cooperation with the Aloe industry. So, Aloe remains a folk remedy used internally for arthritis, stomach ulcers, and diabetes, and externally, for a plethora of skin ailments.

Science:
Beginning to unlock the mystery of Aloe
Aloe contains 146 known constituents that fall into seven basic categories: polysaccharides, anthraquinones, enzymes, fatty acids, amino acids, vitamins, and minerals. In these groups of phytochemicals lie the actives that may help explain the reasons people have been using Aloe for 4000 years.

The anthraquinones in the bitter latex part of the leaf yield the cathartic action of Aloe drug. The polysaccharide constituents exhibit antiviral and immunopotentiating activity. Specifically, acemannan has been documented to enhance the immune system by stimulating the production of macrophages, interferon, lymphocytes, and phagocytic white blood cells. The mucilaginous gel is responsible for Aloe's moisturizing powers, and contains salicylates, which possess anti-inflammatory properties and help to debride a wound of necrotic tissue.

Enzymes in Aloe produce anti-inflammatory and analgesic effects by inactivating bradykinin, a vasodilator involved in immune chemistry. The mineral magnesium lactate blocks the formation of histamine which, when released, causes mucous membranes to swell. And, the essential fatty acid, gamma-linolenic acid (GLA), exerts a favorable effect on inflammation, allergy, platelet aggregation and wound healing, in addition to inhibiting something called thromboxane. Thromboxane is a protein which, released by injured cells as they die, invades the surrounding area, effectively killing adjacent cells.

What else does Aloe do?

Some of the actions that clinical studies have documented are as follows:

> ➢ Even when being rubbed gently onto the skin's surface, Aloe has an amazing ability to penetrate the skin.

> ➢ It appears to slow down the emptying of the stomach and to inhibit the release of excess hydrochloric acid and the enzyme pepsin.

> ➢ Aloe increases tissue levels of several glycosaminoglycans. Glycosaminoglycans are skin components that influence wound healing. They prevent blood clotting, regulate inflammatory cell function, and form a scaffold for the collagen and elastic fibers that knit skin together.

> ➢ It has been shown to improve wound healing in diabetics by either lowering blood glucose levels or by stimulating the function of fibroblasts, the cells that make collagen.

> ➢ Aloe appears to block hydrocortisone's inhibitory effect on wound healing.

> ➢ When given with the drug glyburide, Aloe was shown to improve blood sugar levels when the drug given alone, to the same patient, had not been effective.

Modern Day Uses:

While some claims attributed to Aloe are anecdotal, I believe that enough evidence exists to be comfortable with the use of Aloe Vera, externally as a topical gel, for any of the following:

> ➢ Minor burns

> ➢ Radiation burns
> ➢ Sunburn
> ➢ Windburn
> ➢ Minor cuts
> ➢ Frostbite
> ➢ General skin irritation
> ➢ Wound healing
> ➢ Abrasions
> ➢ Inflammation
> ➢ Itching
> ➢ Acne
> ➢ Increase rate of healing after dental procedures
> ➢ Psoriasis
> ➢ Insect bites and stings
> ➢ Fever blisters
> ➢ Diaper rash
> ➢ Razor burns
> ➢ Bed sores

Internally, Aloe preparations that contain the anthraquinone-laden latex of the plant are potent stimulant laxatives.

Other claims for the oral use of Aloe, many of which do not have strong medical evidence supporting clinical application, include the following:

> ➢ Asthma
> ➢ Peptic ulcers
> ➢ AIDS
> ➢ Arthritis
> ➢ Bursitis
> ➢ Cancer
> ➢ Colitis
> ➢ Diabetes

Dose:

A problem in taking Aloe is that different products vary widely in how much Aloe they actually contain. Manufacturers are not required to list a product's Aloe content. And, when a medicine is 99% water and 1% actives, it is almost impossible to catch cheaters because laboratory tests come back reporting "trace plant materials" present for any Aloe liquid preparation. Purchase your Aloe products from someone you trust.

Topically, apply freely as need. Sometimes I recommend transferring Aloe juice to a plastic spray bottle that can be purchased at the market. This allows one to spray sunburns freely without having to touch the sensitive skin.

For treating the burns of radiation, I actually favor purchasing a great big fat plant or two and harvesting the leaves. Filet them fresh and apply the thick slimy gel directly to the burns.

Internally, I usually recommend a 1-ounce "shooter" before meals. This can be followed with a little water to wash down the bitter Aloe taste. Keep in mind, if your Aloe tastes too good, something might be fishy. Aloe has a distinct taste, and it should be present to ensure you're not getting a watered down version. You can, however, choose to refrigerate it to cut down what your tongue will taste.

An alternative to having to drink Aloe is to find a freeze dried capsule, prepared only from the inner leaf's gel, hence containing no an-thraquinones, or laxative properties. Capsules are available that are standardized to contain the equivalence of 1 ounce of freshly squeezed juice.

Cautions:

Although rarely, topically applied Aloe preparations have been know to cause mild allergic reactions. And, many times preservatives are used that can trigger allergic reactions.

It should be noted that while Aloe is considered a wound healer, it has been shown to actually delay the healing of deep surgical wounds. Aloe actually causes the dermal layer to fuse too quickly, inhibiting the wound from healing properly.

Anthraquinone-containing Aloe products may cause severe gastric cramping and should not be used by pregnant women or children. Additionally, all cautions applicable to any laxative should be heeded.

References:

See General Resources

Atherton, P. "Aloe Vera Revisited." *British Journal of Phytotherapy.* 4:176-83

Ernst, E. "The Clinical Efficacy of Herbal Treatments: An Overview of Recent Systematic Reviews." *The Pharmaceutical Journal,* 1999; 262: 85-87

Ghannam, N. et al. "Antidiabetic Activity of Aloes: Preliminary Clinical and Experimental Observations." *Hormone Research.* 1986; 24:288-94

Hamilton, R. "Strengths and Limitations of Aloe Vera." *American Journal of Natural Medicine.* 1998; 5:30-33

Heggers, J. et al. "Beneficial Effects of Aloe in Wound Healing." *Phytotherapy Res.* 1987; 7:S48-S52

Journal of Ethnopharmacology. 1998; 58:179-86 and 59:195-201

Syed, T. et al. "Management of Psoriasis With Aloe Vera Extract in a Hydrophylic Cream: A Placebo-Controlled, Double-Blind Study." *Tropical Medicine and International Health.* 1996 1:505-09

Astragalus

(Astragalus membranaceous)

Other Common Names:
Huang-Qi, Huang Chi, Milk Vetch

Background:
Astragalus comes to us from Traditional Chinese Medicine (TCM), where it is first mentioned in Shen Nung Ben Cao Jing, a 2000- year-old classic as *Huang Qi*. *Huang Qi* means "yellow leader," and astragalus is considered a most important tonic. Traditional uses include lethargy, colds, flu, appetite (lack of), stomach ulcers, and deficiencies of *chi* (namely, general weakness and fatigue). Other Chinese uses include diabetes, lowering blood pressure, and water retention.

The plant is native to northern China where the 4-7 year old roots are harvested in the spring to make medicine preparations. There are over 2000 types of Astragalus worldwide, but it seems that the Chinese variety has been the most studied. Astragalus gummifera, also known as tragacangth, is an old friend of the pharmaceutical industry, long used as a thickening agent.

Widely known as an energy tonic in China, Astragalus is fast becoming as well known in the West as an immune strengthening agent, or what the Chinese call "protective energy."

Science:
The root of Astragalus contains a long list of tongue twisting phytochemicals. Of note are a series of cycloartane triterpene glycosides called astragalosides, a variety of polysaccharides with names like astragalen, and isoflavone glycosides, which some manufactures use as a standardizing chemical despite reports of biological activity. A typical standard should be not less than .4% 4-hydorxy 3-methoxyisoflavone.

Based on clinical observations, Astragalus' phytoactives have been shown to stimulate the growth of isolated human lymphocytes, potentiate immunological responses, and increase phagocytosis. In cells from cancer patients, which were resistant to immunostimulation, an Astragalus extract increased defense components called mononuclear cells (macrophages and lymphocytes).

Modern Day Uses:

Current interest, while not limited to, are centered around Astragalus' adaptogenic and immune building qualities. The Chinese use it as a classic energy tonic, often in place of Ginseng for people under 40 years of age. Many TCM experts find Ginseng may be too stimulating for younger adults. I guess us old farts can just hold our Ginseng a little better.

My greatest interest in Astragalus is its immune boosting action. Good Western research has pointed to Astragalus' ability to restore normal immune function in cancer patients. Data suggests that patients undergoing chemo or radiotherapies recover faster and live longer if given Astragalus.

A second front that Astragalus may show value in is for HIV infection. Chinese studies with formulae containing Astragalus root found improvements in subjective measures and symptomatology. I am always guarded against offering false hope, but future and larger studies will help guide uses in this area, in addition to the treatment of myasthenia gravis.

I personally use an Astragalus-containing Chinese resistance builder during the cold and flu season. While not considered an herb for acute illness, Astragalus nonetheless is a valuable "wellness" botanical.

Dose:

Many forms of Astragalus are available commercially. Most standardized extracts call for doses of 500mg two to three times daily. Dried root preparations might require dosages upwards of 4 grams daily.

Cautions:

None known.

References:

See General Resources

Cancer Research. 1988; 48:1410-5

Lu, W. "Prospect for Study on Treatment of AIDS with Traditional Chinese Medicine. *J Trad Chin Med* 1995; 15:3.

Sun Y, et al. "Immune Restoration and/or Augmentation of Local Graft vs. Host Reaction by Traditional Chinese Medicinal Herbs." *Cancer.* 1983; 52:70

Tang W, et al. Chinese Drugs of Plant Origin. Berlin: Springer-Verlag, 1992

Wang, Z et al. "Studies on the Chemical Constituents of Astragalus." *Chung Tsao Yao.* 1983; 14:97-99

Zhang, Z, et al. *Journal of Ethnopharmacology*, Sept. 1990

Bilberry

(Vaccinium myrtillus)

Other Common Names:

Whortleberry, Blueberry, Burren Myrtle, Dyeberry, Huckleberry, Hurtleberry, Wineberry, Black Whortles, Hurts, Bleaberry, Airelle, Trackleberry

Background:

Bilberry is a small shrub that grows in the hills and mountains of Europe, Asia and North America. A relative of our Blueberry, Bilberry has been around as a medicinal plant going back to 16th century Europe.

Both the leaves and the fruit of Bilberry have been used as medicines. The leaves remain primarily a folk remedy and do not seem nearly as important as the fruit has become. They have been prepared essentially as teas and used for their astringent, tonic, anti-inflammatory and antiseptic qualities. The leaves have also been shown to have a weak hypoglycemic effect and have been used in various concoctions as treatment for diabetes.

Elizabethan apothecaries made a syrup of the berries with honey, called *Rob*, to treat diarrhea. The fruit, also made as a type of tea and prepared by cooking rather than steeping, has been used to remedy diarrhea, as a diuretic, and as a nutritive to treat scurvy. Dried and ground berries have been used to treat vomiting. But, it wasn't until Word War II that Bilberry became glorified.

As the story goes, the responsibility of bombing Germany was divided between the American and British Royal Air Force. Since night vision equipment was not yet in use, the American Air Force opted for the day shift, so they could see what they were doing in. The Brits got stuck with night raids.

Had there been night vision goggles during Word War II, medicine might be missing one of its great botanicals today. RAF pilots reported improved eyesight after having Bilberry jam and tea prior to their night flying missions over Europe and so made this a regular snack before missions. In the 1960s, based on these stories, Italian and French scientists began researching the berries for their visual benefits.

Science:

The leaves contain a component call glucoquinine. This phytochemical has experimentally been shown to lower blood sugar, hence the basis for diabetic teas used in folk remedies. German researchers believe Bilberry has potential, based on its quinic acid content, for the treatment of gout and rheumatism. However, it is the berries, and specifically their flavonoid compounds know as anthocyanosides, which give Bilberry its claim to fame.

The activity of Bilberry is related to, almost entirely, its anthocyanoside content, as research has primarily keyed on it. The concentration of anthocyanosides in fresh fruit is about .1% to .25%, whereas the concentrated extracts of Bilberry, with which the research has been done, come in at 32-38%. Since the fruit has such a low content, I have to wonder just how much jam those Brits had to eat before they flew. And, since the fruit can have a laxative effect, I wonder what else they were bombing. Nevertheless, for scientific purposes, the anthocyanoside content is expressed specifically as anthocyanidin, and the standardized level of an extract should not be less than is 25%.

Bilberry's anthocyanosides strengthen connective tissue and promote collagen synthesis. They posses potent antioxidant free radical scavenging powers, and they reduce the release of inflammatory chemicals in the body. These actions are consistent with procyanidines found in grapeseed and pine bark extracts and should also help the health of tendons, ligaments, and cartilage.

Anthocyanosides have strong vitamin "P" activity. That is they decrease capillary permeability and fragility. This action is believed to be achieved by an increase in collagen cross-links. Bilberry may have a place in the treatment of vascular disorders including bruising, blood purpuras, ulcerative dermatitis, and varicose veins.

Another effect attributed to the anthocyanoside content of Bilberry is the inhibition of platelet aggregation, making it a cardiovascular protector. The anthocyanoside, myrtillin, has hypoglycemic activity, which may again go to the long history of folk use in the treatment of diabetes. Anthocyanoside extracts may have a smooth muscle relaxing effect, making Bilberry a possible remedy for menstrual cramps. And, they have a protective gastric effect without influencing acid secretion. It is believed that this is achieved by causing the gastric mucosal release of prostaglandin E2. This could block the GI degradation caused by many drugs, or be an ulcer treatment.

Modern Day Uses:

While Bilberry appears to have so many possible uses, I believe the key to its present popularity is due to its affinity for the retina and its potential effects on ophthalmic disorders, namely basic vision, night vision, cataracts, macular degeneration and diabetic retinopathy.

Bilberry extract seems to extend benefit to the eyes by its ability to enhance the supply of blood and oxygen to the eye, in addition to acting as an oxidant. Numerous clinical trials, which included airline pilots, air-traffic controllers, truck drivers, computer operators, navigators, and others, point to significant improvement in eyesight and eyestrain. Bilberry helps the eyes adapt more quickly to darkness and light by stimulating the production of rhodopsin (visual purple) in the retina of the eye. Additionally, a reduction in capillary fragility and hemorrhaging can help alleviate damage to the capillaries in the retina, which is characteristic or retinopathies. Bilberry anthocyanosides may also positively affect eye disorders by enhancing crucial enzymes in retinal cellular metabolism, namely glucose-6phosphatase and phosphoglucomutase.

Dose:

Given the importance of anthocyanosides, I would choose a Bilberry preparation that has been standardized to no less than 25% anthocyanidin. The optimal dose depends on the severity of the condition being treated and whether that condition is acute or chronic.

I would begin a regimen of about 500mg daily divided into two doses.

Some health professionals like three divided doses, but if two better assures your compliance, do it. If significant improvement is achieved, or your interest is only the prevention of eye or circulation problems, consider about 250mg daily.

For best results, use Bilberry extract for 6-8 weeks before evaluating any long-term benefits. If you want to use Bilberry for occasional eyestrain, many people perceive (pun intended) fairly quick results. For those interested in Bilberry strictly for bombing raids, you're on your own.

Cautions:

Bilberry is an extremely safe herb, and there are no known side effects at maintenance or therapeutic doses. Even ridiculously high doses administered to test animals (which I am sorry about), were devoid of toxic effects, with excess blood levels being quickly excreted by the liver and kidney.

However, there are a couple of common sense issues to mention. Bilberry has the ability to decrease platelet aggregation. This may affect clotting times. If you are on medication to thin your blood, discuss your options with your physician so that everybody in alerted.

Since components of Bilberry may have a blood sugar lowering effect, if you are taking diabetic medication, or if you are using insulin, pay attention.

References:

See General Resources

Ann. Med. Accidents Traffic, 3-4, 1965

Australian Journal of Medical Herbalism. Vol. 5. Issue 4, Dec 1993

Bioche*m. Pharmacol.* 32:1141-8, 1983

Christen W. "Antioxidants and Eye Disease." *American Journal of Medicine.* 1994; 97:14S-17S; Discussion, 22S-28S

Cluzel C et al. "Activites Enzymatiques de la Retine et Anthocyanosides Extraits de Vaccinium Myrtillus. *Biochem Pharm."*1970; 19: 2295

Cluzel C, et al. "Activities Phospholglucomustasique et Glucose-6-phosphatasique de la Retine et Anthocyanosides Extraits de Vaccinium Myrtillus." *C.R. Soc. Biol.* 1969; 163:147

Gaz. Med. De France, 18, 25 June 1968

Kadar, A. "Anthocyanosides and Capillary Fragility." *Arterial Wal.* 1979; 5:187-91

Lietti A and Forni G. "Studies on Vaccinium Myrtillus Anthocyanosides." *Arzeimi Hel-Forsch.* 1976; 26:832-835

Mertz-Nielsen A, et al. "A Natural Flavonoid, IdB 1027, Increases Gastric Luminal Release of Prostaglandin E2 in healthy subjects." *Ital J Gastroenterol.* 1990; 22:288

Ophtha*lmology*. 1985; 92:628-635

Rev. Med Aero Spat., 6,5, 1967

Scharrer A and Ober M. "Anthocyanosides in the Treatment of Retinopathies." *Klin Monatsbl Augenheikd.* 1981; 178:386-389

Zaragoza F, et al. "Comparison of Thrombocyte Anti-aAggregant Effects of Anthocyanosides with those of other Agents." *Arch Pharmacol.* 1985; 11:183-188

Black Cohosh

(Cimicifuga racemosa)

Other Common Names:
Black Snakeroot, Squawroot, Rattleroot, Baneberry, Bugbane, Bugroot, Rattleweed, Richweed

Background:
The bug-repellent of medicine?
Black Cohosh is an excellent decorative plant with attractive flowers. It grows in most temperate zones of the Northern Hemisphere, namely Europe, North Asia, North America, and parts of Siberia. It grows wild and is commercially harvested in the region bordered by Canada, Georgia, Arkansas and Wisconsin. For those who want to hunt down some fresh material, look at the edges of woods, in clearings and on riverbanks, if you can handle the consequences. Medicinal plant material comes from cut and dried rootstock, harvested after the fruit has appeared. The reason for using dry root is the unappetizing odor of the fresh plant. Insects even avoid it. In fact, the botanical name of Black Cohosh is Cimicifuga. It comes from the Latin *cimex*, meaning bug, and *fuga*, meaning to repel, hence, bug-repellent.

Black Cohosh was used by North American Indian medicine men for various symptoms, depending on the time of day the root was harvested. They used it as an antidote for poison and snakebite, kidney ailments, malaria, rheumatism, sore throat, and various female problems, hence the name "Squawroot."

Early American colonists, who probably learned from our native Americans, found Black Cohosh useful for upper respiratory problems, malaria, nervous disorders, and yellow fever.

In the early 1800s, it was used by the Eclectic Physicians to treat muscular pain associated with rheumatism, menstrual problems, radiating pain of neuralgia, and inflammation. It was also used to treat consumption and for its ability to lower blood pressure. Actually, it was an official drug of the U.S. Pharmacopoeia from 1820 to 1926.

If there are any old-timers reading this, they might remember Lydia Pinham's Vegetable Compound. It contained Black Cohosh and was one of the most prominent women's tonics on the market from the early 1900s into the 1950s. But it wasn't until 1944 that von Gizycki discovered Black cohosh's estrogen-like effect.

Hormone replacement therapy (HRT) is a very big and controversial business in this country. Estrogen is regularly prescribed for the normal simple process of menopause, while its link to increased cancer incidence seems to be played down or covered up. I find it interesting to note that studies of HRT, which are mostly European, estimate an up to 13 fold increase in endometrial cancer risk, and an up 30% increase in breast cancer risk, while only a few studies in the United States show HRT increases cancer. Something seems fishy.

Although many hormone replacement therapies employed today are less aggressive, they are still far from risk free. Many physicians will not even prescribe estrogen for women with a history of cancer, unexplained uterine bleeding, liver or gall bladder disorders, stroke, heart attack, blood clots, uterine fibroid tumors, or fibrocystic breast disease. These are some key reasons why Black Cohosh is so heavily prescribed in Europe, and becoming increasingly more popular in the U.S.

A safe phytoestrogen

Estrogen is actually estrogens, not just one, but three different hormone fractions. The primary estrogen, *estradiol*, is the fraction most associated with an increase in breast, ovarian, and endometrial cancer risk. On the other hand, *estriol*, another estrogen, is actually associated with some protection against cancer. Not all estrogens are bad. The reason *estriol* is good is that it has a much weaker action than the other two estrogens, with a shorter dwelling time on receptors. Estrogen-fed tumors are not stimulated by *estriol*, the weak sister, which also competes for available estrogen receptor sites and thus acts as a partial antagonist to *estradiol*, the big mean sibling. Black Cohosh contains phytochemicals which allow it to be considered an estriol-like phytoestrogen, but before we herbalize Cinderella, let's move on.

Science:

The most medically valuable constituents of Black Cohosh are called triterpenoid glycosides. While many alcohol, full spectrum, extracts are used in Europe successfully, the core of impressive clinical studies have utilized an extract, standardized to 2.5% triterpene glycoside, measured as 27-deoxyaceteine. And, these controlled studies suggest that Black Cohosh, delivering 4 mg of 27-deoxyaceteine, produces symptomatic relief of menopausal symptoms comparable to HRT, but without the risk of serious side effects.

Triterpenoids do not alone make Black Cohosh a valuable plant. Like almost all phytomedicines, Black Cohosh is a blend of many active constituents. In addition to the glycosides acetin and cimicfugoside, it contains aromatic acids, tannins, resins, fatty acids, and isoflavones, paramount of which is formononetin.

It is the formononetin that is believed to bind to estrogen receptor sites, thus inducing an estrogen-like effect. The triterpenoids, on the other hand, work on the hypothalamus-pituitary axis. You see, as meno-pause comes on, estrogen and progesterone levels drop. In response to this, the pituitary increases the release of two other hormones called follicle-stimulating hormone (FSH) and luteinizing hormone (LH). It is the increase in LH levels that affects the vasomotor activity that is responsible for some or the more obnoxious menopausal symptoms like hot flashes and night sweats. Black Cohosh, with its triterpenoids, has been shown to lower LH. Very cool stuff.

Modern Day Uses:

Based on clinical studies and the experience of over 1.5 million women, Black Cohosh looks like an effective alternative to hormone replacement therapy. It has proven itself effective for physical meno-pausal symptoms including hot flashes, night sweats, headaches, heart palpitations, and vaginal atrophy; and psychological symptoms includ-ing depression, anxiety, nervousness, sleep disturbances, and decreased libido.

Studies indicate that Black Cohosh can relieve menopausal symptoms to a similar extent to estriol, conjugated estrogens, and estrogen/

progestin sequential therapy. It did not stimulate estrogen-dependent breast tumor cells in cell culture studies and may be a good alternative to HRT for women at risk for breast cancer or patient populations with a history of estrogen-dependent cancer. On the contrary, one might expect to see inhibitory activity.

Additionally, Black Cohosh exerts no action on the endometrium of the uterus. Therefore, it is not necessary to oppose therapy with progesterone like you do in conventional HRT.

Other uses of Black Cohosh include PMS, dysmenorrhea, hypercholesteremia, and peripheral arterial disease as well as many of the historical indications our forefathers (and mothers) used it for.

Dose:
If you are a holistic type, take a whole herb preparation, 500mg three times daily. However, if you want to be consistent with the most recent, intensive, and successful clinical evidence, take an extract standardized to 2.5% triterpene glycoside, measured as, and yielding 1-2 mg of 27-deoxyaceteine. Take the equivalent of 2mg 27-deoxyaceteine twice daily. Allow 4 weeks for maximum effects to take hold.

While HRT is intended to be used long term, Black Cohosh does not have to be. It is generally used to help the patient through the symptom stages of menopause. The average length that one might take Black Cohosh for is 6-18 months.

Cautions:
Aside from rare stomach upset, there are no known side effects. There are no known drug interactions. And again, according to the German FDA, actually called the BGA, there are no contraindications or limitations of use in tumor patients or any of the limitations to hormone replacement use (see above). Therefore, Black Cohosh is considered a suitable natural alternative to HRT, especially where HRT is not an option.

Black Cohosh should, however, be avoided during pregnancy or if lactating, unless being used under the care of a health care professional.

References:

See General Resources

Beuscher, N. "Cimicifuga Racemosa L." *Zeitschrift fur Phytotherapie*. 1995; 16:301-310

Brinker, F. "Macrotys." *The Eclectic Medical Journals*. 1996; Feb/Mar: 2-4

DerMarderosian, A ed. *Review of Natural Products*. St. Louis, MO, Facts and Comparisons, 1999

Duke, J. *Handbook of Medicinal Herbs*. Boca Ratan FL, CRC Press Inc., 1985

Krochmal, A. and Krochmal, C. *A Guide to the Medicinal Plant of United States*. New York, Quadrangle/The New York Times Book Co. 1975

Liske, E, Duker, E. "Cimicifuga Racemosa in Clinical Practice and Research. *Ars Medici*. 1993 7:1-8

Schultz V, Hansel, R, Tyler, V. *Rational Phytotherapy: A Physician's Guide to Herbal Medicine*. Heidelberg, Germany, Springer Verlag, 1998

Butcher's Broom

(Ruscus aculeatus)

Other Common Names:

Kneeholy, Knee Holly, Kneeholm, Jew's Myrtle, Sweet Broom, Pettigree, Box Holly

Background:

The medicinal use of Butcher's Broom dates back some 2,000 years to classical Greece where it was prescribed as a laxative and diuretic. It is one the herbs that didn't do much to contribute to botanical medicine until this century. The 1950s uncovered clinical evidence of Butcher's Broom's vein-toning activity and its potential value in the treatment of circulatory diseases.

The name Knee Holly is, like many common names for plants, descriptive, as this botanical grows about knee high and has prickly leaves like a true Holly. I am sure that walking through a field of these would probably get your attention.

The young shoot of Butcher's Broom used to be eaten much like Asparagus, a related plant. But, its most famous use, until modern times, has been as a broom used by butchers to sweep their blocks. They would collect matured leaves and bind them into bundles for sweeping.

Science:

Butcher's Broom as a medicine is extracted from both the roots and the above ground portions of the plant. The primary components of the extract are isolated from the plant's steroidal saponins. The significant ingredients are ruscogenin and neoruscogenin. Better extracts are standardized to ruscogenin.

Both animal and human studies suggest that Butcher's Broom may be of benefit in the management of venous insufficiency. In one study, it was shown to be effective in improving the effects of lower limb venous disease in patients with chronic disease. Symptoms including swelling, itching, tingling, limb heaviness, and cramping were greatly improved.

Modern Day Uses:
Possible uses of Butcher's Broom or herbal combinations that contain Butcher's Broom include:

> ➤ Leg edema and cramps
> ➤ Varicose veins
> ➤ Peripheral vascular disease
> ➤ Hemorrhoids
> ➤ Painful veins
> ➤ Frostbite
> ➤ Heavy legs

Dose:
Butcher's Broom is generally used in herbal blends formulated for circulation. Choose a formula that delivers at least 100 to 150 mg daily of Butcher's Broom, standardized to a minimum of 10% saponins (as ruscogenin). You might also consider taking a tablet of vitamin C with bioflavonoids with your Butchers Broom. This is how one of the clinical trials was performed.

Cautions:
None known.

References:
See General Resources

Capelli, R. et al. "Use of Extract of Ruscus Aculeatus in Venous Disease in the Lower Limbs." *Drugs Exp Clin Res*. 1988; 14:277-83

Rubanyi, G. et al. "Effect of Temperature on the Responsiveness of Cutaneous Veins the Extract of Ruscus aculeatus." *Gen Pharmacl*. 1984; 15:431

Tyler, V et al. *Pharmacognosy*. 9th ed. Philadelphia, PA. Lea & Febiger. 1988

Weiner, M. *Weiner's Herbal*. Mill Valley. CA. Quantum Books.

Cascara Sagrada

(Rhamnus purshiana)

Other Common Names:

Cascara, Buckthorn, Chittem Bark, Sacred Bark, Holy Bark, Christ's Thorn, Bearberry Tree, Bearwood, Persiana Bark, Persian Bark, Brittle Wood, Polecat Tree, Coffee Berry

Background:

Cascara is a deciduous tree that grows from 20 to 40 feet high. The part used in herbal medicine is the bark. The bark is what holds the active principles of Cascara, and these chemicals are so potent that the bark must be aged for at least one year to temper its force. Cascara is a laxative, and fresh bark would produce too strong an effect and could induce vomiting.

Cascara trees are found on the sides and bottoms of canyons from the Rocky Mountains to the Pacific Ocean, and from California to British Columbia. Native Americans originally introduced early Spanish priests in California to the value of Cascara, which may account for some of its common names.

Cascara came into mainstream medicinal use in 1877 when an Eclectic physician, Dr. J.H. Bundy wrote about it. The Detroit-based pharmaceutical company, Parke-Davis & Company began marketing it, and it became an officially listed drug of the U.S. Pharmacopoeia in 1890. Cascara is still used in over-the-counter laxatives throughout the country in pharmacies. One of the few herbals to weather the changing times.

Science:

The laxative properties of Cascara are due to compounds called anthraquinones. Anthraquinones are common to other natural laxatives like Aloe and Senna, but in the case of Cascara, they are special anthracene glycosides called Cascarosides A and B. Cascarosides make up about two-thirds of the plants' anthraquinones, and good quality product should not have less than 60-70%. Anthraquinones act on the large intestine to induce peristaltic waves and hence evacuation.

Cascara's Cascarosides act by producing water and electrolyte secretion in the small intestine and inhibiting these secretions in the large intestine. The net effect is an increase of volume in the bowel, the swelling of which stimulates expulsion. And, with Cascara, this action is exerted with a minimum of stimulant laxative side effects.

Modern Day Uses:
Cascara is indicated anytime a mild laxative may be necessary:

> ➢ Chronic or acute constipation
> ➢ Hemorrhoids
> ➢ Anal fissures
> ➢ Post rectal-anal surgery
> ➢ To restore tone to the colon and overcome laxative dependence in the elderly
> ➢ Detoxification and cleansing programs

Some herbalists also prescribe Cascara in small doses, both as a liver tonic and as a chelating agent to prevent calcium-based urinary stones.

Dose:
Depending on the concentration of actives, it is best to follow the manufacturer's instructions. Generally speaking, one or two 500mg capsules daily is adequate. Laxative action is usually seen within six to eight hours, so plan ahead.

Cascara can appropriately be used for children over two years of age. Follow the guidelines prepared by the manufacturer. The recommended dosage will probably be ¼ to ½ the adult dose.

Cautions:
Because Cascara crosses the placental barrier and is excreted in breast milk, it should be avoided during pregnancy and breast-feeding. Use bulk-forming laxatives instead.

Chronic use or abuse of any laxative can lead to electrolyte imbalances, especially potassium depletion. This can create serious problems if one is taking certain kinds of heart, or blood pressure medicines.

Laxatives should not be used by people with intestinal obstruction or inflammation. That means that if you have Crohn's disease, colitis, appendicitis, or abdominal pain of unknown origin, don't use laxatives.

References:

See General Resources

DerMarderosian, A ed. *Review of Natural Products*. St. Louis, MO, Facts and Comparisons, 1999

Rhamnus purshiana cortex. ESCOP. Monograph, 1997

Lloyd, J, et al. *Kings American Dispensatory*. 18th ed. Portland, OR, Eclectic Medical Publications. 1983

Cat's Claw

(Uncaria tomentosa)

Other Common Names:

Una de Gato, Samento, Rangaya, Garabato, Unganangui, Life Giving Vine of Peru

Background:

Cat's Claw is a woody vine that winds itself around trees, upwards of 100 feet, in the Peruvian rainforests. Hook-like thorns adorn the leaves, resembling the claws of cats, hence the name. For hundreds of years, local Indians, medicine people, and shamans have stewed the inner bark and roots of Cat's Claw to prepare medicines to treat a variety of illnesses.

There are actually over 30 species of Uncaria, however the two species of medicinal interest are U. guianensis and U. tomentosa. Although both species produce similar benefits, U. tomentosa has been more thoroughly researched, has a greater range of uses, and is hence pre-ferred in the American market.

In researching the benefits of Cat's Claw, the only thing I couldn't find its consumption good for is the loose spokes on my bicycle rims, and I can't say for sure it's not good for that too. Here is a partial list of ailments that Cat's Claw is purported to benefit: arthritis, cancer, fibromyalgia, lupus, respiratory infections, allergies, shingles, prostate problems, asthma, rheumatism, viral infections, diverticulitis, colitis, leaky gut syndrome, menstrual problems, a contraceptive, acne, de-pression, gonorrhea, diabetes, hypoglycemia, parasites, candida, intestinal flora imbalances, gastritis, ulcers, Crohn's disease, hemor-rhoids, herpes, AIDS, cirrhosis, chronic fatigue syndrome, multiple sclerosis, and the ill effects of radiation and chemotherapy.

Whether or not these purported benefits will all stand up to scientific scrutiny is yet to be seen. We can only hope that appropriate research will continue. In the meantime, some clinical evidence does exist. In fact, scientific studies by the National Cancer Institute have verified both anticancer and immune stimulating properties of Cat's Claw.

Science:

Cat's Claw, like most plants, is extremely complex in its composition and is very rich in phytochemical actives. Research has uncovered a host of chemical components that may very well explain its folkloric uses.

The active constituents that appear to be the most important are a group of alkaloids called oxindole alkaloids. These oxindoles include isopteropodine, pteropodine, isomitraphylline, rhynchophylline, isorynchophylline, and mytraphylline. Four of these components have been found to have profound immunostimulating properties. Isopteropodine is the most active of these. In fact, researchers use it, in addition to total oxindole alkaloids, as the standard determining the quality of Una de Gato.

A recent study has suggested that there are two chemotypes of the plant. Each chemotype has a different oxindole alkaloid pattern. One type has a greater tetracyclic oxindole level, the other a greater pentacyclic oxindole level. This ratio may be significant. The study claims that it is the penacyclic fraction that has the immunomodulating effect on cells, and the tetracyclic fraction antagonizes this action of the pentacyclics. Questions still remain to be answered, and I am looking for more studies to be published. This one looks like it was sponsored by an Austrian company that is the patent holder on the process of extracting this new Cat's Claw chemotype. They also have a product on the market.

The oxindole, Rhynchophylline, may have significant cardiovascular properties. It has been shown to inhibit platelet aggregation and thrombosis. It has been suggested that this phytochemical may be useful in reducing the risk of heart attack by lowering blood pressure, increasing circulation and by preventing the formation of blood clots.

Oxindole alkaloids are not the only components of Cat's Claw that are of medicinal value. The plant also contains quinovic glycosides, triterpines, polyphenols, proanthocyanidines, and phytosterols. The quinovic acid glycosides in Una de Gato have been shown to display anti-viral actions. Triterpines show anti-viral, anti-ulcer, antioxidant , anti-inflammatory, anti-allergic, and increased killer cell activity. Polyphenols and proanthocyanidines, like those found in grapeseed, green tea, and other various fruits and vegetables are powerful antioxidants. And, phytosterols help control cholesterol and can act as hormone precursors that can possess anti-tumor and anti-inflammatory properties.

Now, take all this science and apply it back to South America's history of folkloric uses.

Modern Day Uses:
With the wealth of possible benefits Cat's Claw might offer, where does it fit in modern uses? Well, two primary areas that cannot be ignored are immune stimulation and anti-inflammatory action. Studies within the last decade have confirmed these activities.

It is generally recognized that Cat's Claw can enhance the process of phagocytosis, that is, the process by which our immune system engulfs and destroys invaders and mutations. Reports have demonstrated that it can improve immunity in cancer patients, and act as an anti-mutagenic, and anti-viral agent. Additionally, given the aforementioned, in light of the fact that Cat's Claw has been used to reduce the side effects of radiation and chemotherapy in conventional cancer treatments, there seems to be a foundation upon which to marry the treatments.

And, while strong clinical evidence of Una de Gato's usefulness in treating systemic inflammatory and inflammatory gastrointestinal diseases seems to be lacking, its reported value for the treatment of arthritis, rheumatism, diverticulitis, gastritis, Crohn's disease, dysentery, and ulcers cannot be ignored.

Other interesting uses are under current study. Cat's Claw is being used in some studies in combination with AZT to both slow the progression of AIDS, and to reduce the drug's side effects. Additionally, Peruvian research has demonstrated positive effects in treating children with leukemia. Studies on cats with leukemia are also underway.

Dose:

In terms of dosage, since this is an herbal medicine that has generally been used in a crude form, namely a decoction, a brew of bark and leaves, perhaps it makes more sense to use a full spectrum extract rather than a substance concentrated to any one component.

Look for an extract somewhere in the neighborhood of 4:1. Meaning that for each 100 grams of crude plant, 25 grams of solids have been extracted. Having found such an extract, take 500mg to 1000mg three times daily.

Cautions:

One of the areas of caution that must be discussed is product quality. Cat's Claw can refer to at least 20 plants from 12 different families, some with a completely different chemical make-up, medicinally unrelated, and some of which have been reported as toxic to humans. They all may go by the name Una de Gato. Couple this with the fact that plants may be harvested by natives living in poverty, some of whom may not be trained in plant identification, and others of whom might not care. There are even rumors of sources in Peru grinding the entire vine and selling a diluted product.

One can only hope that unsuspecting manufacturers in the United States are buying from reputable raw material exporters who are testing plants for positive identification and concentration of actives, and then testing for themselves. There are even seasonal concentration variations to consider, even if the plant material is good.

A few common sense contraindications and interactions should be considered. First are hypotensives. Since Cat's Claw may lower blood pressure, one should use it with caution if using blood pressure medicine already. Monitor your pressure. If it goes down, discuss your options with your primary care physician. Perhaps he or she may want to adjust your drug dose.

Since Cat's Claw has been used in Traditional Peruvian Medicine for birth control and as an abortifacient, it certainly doesn't make sense to use if you are pregnant or trying to get pregnant.

Cat's Claw possesses actives that may naturally thin blood and prevent clotting. This is a good action for most of us, but those who are taking blood-thinning drugs should take note. Discuss the use with your physician. Let he or she monitor your clotting time if you decide to use the herb.

If you are undergoing skin grafts or an organ transplant, beware. Cat's Claw is an immune system stimulant. It will encourage your body to attack foreign bodies.

Even though some may be precluded from using Cat's Claw, published data points to it as having very low toxicity and being quite safe to use.

References:

See General Resources

Success Achieved with Una de Gato in the Fight Against AIDS in Austria. El Comercio. Lima Peru. 1988

Chen, C et al. "Inhibitory Effect of Rhynchophylline on Platelet Aggregation and Thrombosis*." Chung Kuo Yao Li Hsueh Pao* 1992: 13:126-30

Duke, J, Vasquez, R. *Amazonian Ethnobotanical Dictionary*. Boca Raton, FL: CRC Press 1994

Duke, J. Handbook of Medicinal Herbs. Boca Raton, FL: CRC Press, 1985

Hemingway, S, and Philipson, J. "Alkaloids from South American Species of Uncaria." *J Pharm Pharmacol*. 1974; 26:113

Jones, K. "The Herb Report: Una de Gato, Life-Giving Vine of Peru." *Am Herb Assoc* 1994; 10(3):4.

Keplinger, W. "Oxindole Alkaloids Having Properties Stimulating the Immunologic System," US Patent No. 4,844,901, July 1989

Keplinger, K, et al. "Uncaria Tomentosa-Ethnomedical Use and New Pharmacological Toxicological and Botanical Results." 1999; 64:23-34

Maxwell, N. *Witch Doctor's Apprentice*. 3rd edition. New York: Citadel Press 1990

Reinhard, K. "Unaria Tomentosa (Willd.) D.C.: Cat's Claw, Una De Gato, or Saventaro." *The Journal of Alternative and Complementary Medicine*. 5:143-151

Cayenne

(Capsicum annuum; C. frutescens)

Other Common Names:

Capsicum, Red Pepper, African Chilies, Tabasco Pepper, Paprika, Pimiento, Mexican Chilies, Bird Pepper, Capsicum Fruit, Garden Pepper, Goats Pod, Hot Pepper, Hungarian Pepper, Louisiana Long Pepper, Louisiana Sport Pepper, Zanzibar Pepper, Mexican Chili, African Chili, Spanish Pepper, Pod Pepper, Cockspur Pepper, Ginnie Pepper

Background:

One of the oldest cultivated plants known

Cayenne or Capsicum consists of the dried fruit of Capsicum frutescens, Capsicum annum, or a large number of hybrids of these species and varieties within the Solanaceae (Nightshade) family that are capsaicin rich. Because these plants have been cultivated for such a long time, peppers from them differ widely from one another in size, shape, and potency. They are not true peppers but were misnamed by the early Spanish explorers who confused their pungency with the pepper they were used to, namely black pepper (Piper nigrum) in the Piperaceae family.

The Capsicums are ancient natives of the tropical Americas. The oldest known specimens were discovered in Mexico from seeds found on the floors of caves and in ancient fossil feces. From these samples, scientists were able to conclude that these people were eating peppers as far back as 7000 BC They also believe that hot peppers were cultivated between 5200 and 3400 BC, making the capsicum peppers one of the oldest cultivated plants in the world. Chili is the Aztec name for Cayenne pepper.

A Dr. Diego Chanca, the physician who accompanied Christopher Columbus on his second voyage to the West Indies, brought capsicum peppers back to Europe. From Europe, Capsicum found its way to most balmy tropical zones worldwide. When these plants were intro-duced into traditional Indian Ayurvedic medicine, the prototype to the back plasters I can remember my father using when I was a child was invented. In Chinese medicine, cayenne is considered a great digestive stimulant, in addition to being used topically to treat myalgia (muscle pain). In Japan, an alcoholic extract of Cayenne was applied to treat frostbite. Interestingly, I have come across products that I can put into my mountaineering boots as feet warmers that are Capsicum-based.

In 1548, Cayenne was introduced into Britain from India, then known as Ginnie or Guinea pepper because of its cultivation prevalence in this locale. The famous English botanist and barber-surgeon, Gerard, (talented folks did double duty in those days), described it in his classic work, *The Herbal*, as "extreme hot and dry, even in the fourth degree." He recommended it for scrofula, an obsolete term for cervical lymph gland swelling due to tuberculosis. In Gerard's day, scrofula was prevalent and considered a throat disorder known as the King's Evil. Cayenne is still used by some to treat throat problems such as tonsillitis, laryngitis, and hoarseness.

As a folk medicine in parts of Russia, Cayenne is marinated in Vodka and drunk in wineglass doses as a tonic. I know people who do this today by ordering pepper flavored vodka martinis. Either remedy in wineglassful doses probably covers up a multitude of pains.

Pass the sauce
An American banker, returning from the Mexican-American War (1846-1848), brought with him some local pepper seeds. He grew plants from them in Louisiana and found that the peppers made a wonderful spicy sauce. He left Louisiana during the Civil War, and when he returned, he found his plants were one of the few things still flourishing. Since the war left him without a job, he decided to market the delightful sauce he used to make. The venture proved to be a very successful business. The man's name was Edward McIlhenny. The original pepper seeds came from the Mexican state of Tabasco, and his product was, and is, known as Tabasco Sauce.

Once an official medicine
In the United States, Capsicum was an official drug listed in both the U.S. Pharmacopoeia and the National Formulary into the 1950s. It was listed as a carminative (relieves gas), stimulant, and rubefacient

(used as a counterirritatant for muscle pain). Cayenne is still an official drug in Germany approved in the Commission E monographs.

Traditionally Cayenne has been used for its stimulant actions, especially with respect to the circulatory and digestive systems. It is said to
increase blood flow thus allaying peripheral vascular disorders, decrease blood pressure, tonify the nervous system, increase appetite,
relieve indigestion, and act as a carminative (relieves gas and flatulence). It has antiseptic and antibacterial properties and has made for
an excellent gargle for sore throats.

Cayenne can be useful as a diaphoretic (a sweat-inducing herb),
especially when used with Yarrow. Old timers used it at the first onset
of a cold, when a chill was coming on, or to break a fever.

The Chinese believe Cayenne stimulates yang, the masculine active
principle in nature that is exhibited in light, heat, or dryness and that
combines with yin to produce harmony in the body. They also believe,
as do most herbalists, that Cayenne is an accentuator of other herbs,
increasing the value and healing properties of other herbs in a formula
by carrying them to afflicted parts of the body via its ability to stimulate circulation.

Science:

Cayenne or Capsicum gets its name for the Greek *kaptos*, meaning I
bite (no leap of faith here). The origin of the species is buried in
antiquity, but experts believe that all of the varieties of chilies came
from one species. Perhaps this is why sometimes Cayenne is described as being derived from C. annuum, and sometimes from C.
frutescens, and other times from a mixture. For this reason, it makes
more sense to judge a Capsicum medicine by the active to which it is
standardized and its heat units value.

Capsaicin and Scoville Heat Units

Cayenne consists of dried ripe fruits that contain up to 1.5%
capsaicinoids. The major component (about 50%) is capsaicin, upon
which most medicinal preparations are based. However, a system to
determine how hot a pepper is also exists. The system was developed
in 1912, by Wilbur L. Scoville, a pharmacist for the company that

developed a muscle rub which they named Heat®. Scoville would mix ground chili, sugar water, and alcohol to determine the number of units a pepper would score. Today Scoville units are still used, but high performance liquid chromatographs do the testing.

A red bell pepper contains very little capsaicin and gets a zero in Scoville Heat Units. The average jalapeño scores about 5000. A wild pepper called the chiltecpin gets 70,000 to 90,000, and Habañeros earn the top spot coming in at 200,000 Scoville Heat Units; the hottest ever registered being 326,000. Can you imagine biting into one of those babies?

While some medical evidence supports Cayenne's effectiveness in various conditions, including gastrointestinal, high blood pressure, high cholesterol, and blood clotting, overwhelming clinical documentation confirms its topical benefits. Ironically, the burning substance in Cayenne relieves chronic pain, and does so by depleting a chemical called Substance P.

What's Substance P, and how does Cayenne affect it?
Substance P is a neuropeptide that is released from peripheral C type nerve fibers. It mediates the transmission of pain impulses to the spinal cord and on to the brain. For example, inflammation in a joint causes the release of Substance P. This stimulates the release of pain signals to sensory nerves that carry those impulses to the brain via the spinal cord. Now the brain knows that something is going on.

Capsaicin does something that no other known substance does; it selectively depletes Substance P in pain transmission nerves. You see, the initial pain we feel when exposed to red pepper is irritation caused by the release of Substance P. However, the supply of Substance P is eventually depleted, lessening further release, or perhaps production, resulting in fewer pain signals sent to the brain. Depletion of Substance P does not occur immediately, and effective use of a topical preparation requires application four or five times daily for periods of at least four weeks.

Additionally, by virtue of a methoxyphenol ring on the Capsaicin molecule, further pain relief may occur due to interference with two enzymes involved in the inflammatory process, namely lipooxygenase and cyclooxygenase. This action is due to Capsaicin's antioxidant activity.

Modern Day Uses:
Topical

> ➢ Post-herpetic neuralgia: the pain associated with shingles.

> ➢ Post-surgical pain: including post-mastectomy and post amputation.

> ➢ Diabetic neuropathy: sensations of pain, temperature, and pressure, especially in the lower legs and feet.

> ➢ Arthritis: both rheumatoid and osteo.

> ➢ Various other neuropathic and complex pain syndromes.

Oral

> ➢ Stimulant to the digestive system.

> ➢ Circulation and high blood pressure.

> ➢ High cholesterol

> ➢ Reduce blood clotting tendencies by reducing platelet aggregation and increasing fibrinolytic activity

> ➢ Prevention or arteriosclerosis and heart disease

> ➢ Prevention of GI damage when taken ½ hour before aspirin

Another potential use for Capsaicin, administered as a nasal spray, is to treat cluster headaches. These are migraine-like headaches that occur in clusters, with no warning signals, one to three times daily for several days.

Psoriasis has been linked to high levels of Substance P in the skin.

This prompted researchers to try topical Capsaicin as a treatment. After three weeks, significant reductions in redness and scales were observed, suggesting possible Capsaicin utility in this menacing disorder.

Counter-intuitively, research suggests that Capsaicin may protect against peptic ulcers. However, remember that Cayenne exerts an antimicrobial effect, and peptic ulcers are often treated with an antibiotic that goes after the bacteria H. pylori. Additionally, Cayenne has been shown to protect the gastric mucosal membrane against damage from alcohol and aspirin.

Researchers from a major drug company reported that Capsaicin was shown to reduce serious heart arrhythmias and improve cardiac blood flow. While these were animal studies, the results are not too far off folkloric uses.

Dose:
Topically, creams containing .025% to .075% are applied to the affected area three to four times daily. Treatment may need to be continued for upwards of six weeks.

Orally, take 30-120mg three times daily. Look for an indication of standardization to Capsaicin, and how many Scoville Heat Units the raw material evidenced when tested.

Cautions:
Fist and foremost, let's put the notion to bed that eating spicy foods containing red peppers is harmful to the stomach lining. Actually, if anything, the opposite is true. Published studies indicate that individuals eating these foods showed no ill effects when compared to a control group. Researchers concluded that ingesting spices is not associated with GI damage. According to *Drug and Chemical Toxicology*, the toxic dose of Tabasco would come after consuming one-half gallon of very hot sauce. Anyone who would do that, deserves to hurt.

Cayenne has a warming effect on the GI tract due to its circulatory stimulation and activation of gastric secretions. The intensity of these reactions is dose and concentration dependent. Therefore, dose should be adjusted to fit into one's comfort level. What would be a digestive aid to one person, might be upsetting to another.

Topically, Capsicum is an irritant. It's supposed to be. Some people will be more sensitive than others, and some might even experience hypersensitivity reactions like urticaria, a small swelling on the skin like that caused by an insect bite, that usually itches or burns. Capsaicinoids are very irritating to mucosal membranes, and inhalation can cause inflammation in the lungs.

Cayenne has been used as a deterrent for thumb sucking or nail biting in children. I would be concerned over this use as what starts off on fingers can end up in the eyes. For those of you who, like myself, have demonstrated that we are not always the sharpest tool on the bench, and have put their contact lenses in after handling a hot pepper, you know how irritating Capsaicinoids can be to the eyes. This is why they are a common component of many self-defense sprays.

Since Cayenne can have a blood thinning effect, a person taking prescription anticoagulants should have his or her clotting times checked, as the medication may have to be down regulated. Theoretically, if Cayenne can enhance the effectiveness of herbs used concomitantly; it could also affect the metabolism of any drugs. For example, it enhances the absorption of thophylline. It could make sedatives more sedating or increase the excretion rate of any substance metabolized by the liver. While this is only speculative, I mention it to encourage you to heighten your awareness level. Stay in touch with your body and notice any changes that take place.

Capsaicinoids are insoluble in cold water and only slightly soluble in warm water. If you want to get a residue off your body, use vinegar, although I would not use it around the eyes. I have heard that milk may be useful also.

References:

See General Resources

Bernstein, J. et al. "Topical Capsaicin Relieves Chronic Post Herpetic Neuralgia." *J Am Acad Dermatol*. 1987;17:93

D'Alonzo, A. et al. *European J of Pharm*. 1995; 272:269-78

Deal, C. et al. "Treatment of Arthritis with Topical Capsaicin." *Clin Ther*. 1991; 13:383-95

Editorial. "Hot Peppers and Substance P". *Lancet*. 1983;335:1198

Ellis, C. et al. "A Double-Blind Evaluation of Topical Capsaicin in Pruritic Psoriasis." *J Am Acad Dermtol*. 1993; 29:438-442

Horowitz, M. et al. "The Effect of Chili on Gastrointestinal Transit." *J Gastroenterol Hepatol*. 1992;7:52-56

Kang, J. et al. *Gut*, 1995; 36:664-449

Kawada, T. et al. "Effects of Capsaicin on Lipid Metabolism in Rats Fed a High Fat Diet." *J Nutr*. 1986; 116:1272-1278

Lembeck, F. "Columbus, Capsicum and Capsaicin: Past, Present and Future." *Acta Physiol Hung*. 1987;69:265-273

Marks, D. et al. "A Double-Blind Placebo Controlled Trial of Intranasal Capsaicin for Cluster Headache." *Cephalagia*. 1993; 13:114-116

McCarthy, G. et al. "Effect of Topical Capsaicin in the Therapy of Painful Osteoarthritis of the Hands." *J Rheumatol*. 1992; 19:604-7

Monsereenusorn, Y. "Subchronic Toxicity Studies of Capsaicin and Capsicum in Rats." *Res Commun Chem Pathol Pharmacol*. 1983;41:95

Palevitch, D., Craker, L. "Nutritional and Medical Importance of Red Pepper." *J Herbs Spices Med Plants*. 1995;3:55-83

Tandan, R. et al. "Topical Capsaicin in Painful Diabetic Neuropathy." *Diabetes Care*. 1992; 15:15-18

Tyler, V. *Herbs of Choice*. New York. The Haworth Herbal Press. 1999

Yeoh, K, et al. "Chili Protects Against Aspirin-Induced Gastrointestinal mucosal Injury in Humans." *Gif Dis Sci*. 1995; 49;580-3

Watson, C. et al. "The Post-Mastectomy Pain Syndrome and the Effect of Topical Capsaicin." *Pain*.1989; 38:177-186

Watson, C. et al. "Post-Herpetic Neuralgia and Topical Capsaicin." *Pain*. 1988; 35:289-97

Wood, A. "Determination of the Pungent Principles of Chilies and Ginger by Reversed Phase HPLC with Use of a Single Standard Substance." J *Flavour Fragrance*. 1987;2:1-12

Chamomile

(Matricaria recutita)

Other Common Names:

M. recutita: German Chamomile, M. chamomilla, True Chamomile, Wild Chamomile, Hungarian Chamomile, True Chamomile, Genuine Chamomile, Pin Heads, Sweet False Chamomile

Chamaemelum nobile: Roman Chamomile, English Chamomile, Anthemis nobilis, Garden Chamomile, Sweet Chamomile, Ground Apple, Low Chamomile, Whig Plant

Background:

To us in the United States, Chamomile is considered a beverage, generally consumed in the evening. In Europe, it is best known as an herbal medicine. In fact, German Chamomile is listed as a medicine in the pharmacopoeias of 26 countries. It has been said that Chamomile is to Europe what Ginseng is to Asia. In Germany in 1987, Chamomile was designated the plant of the year. This is surprising to me; having been to Germany many times, I would have expected tobacco to be the plant of the year, every year.

The common name, Chamomile, actually refers to two different plants, German Chamomile and Roman Chamomile. German is an annual and Roman is a perennial. Roman is favored by England, and German is much more widely used throughout the rest of the world. The Germans often refer to their Chamomile as Genuine or True Chamomile, and the English often refer to theirs as Common or English Chamomile. Roman Chamomile was not cultivated in Rome until the 16th century, and it probably came from Britain. Would you believe that there are about 24 names to designate these two species? This is why some botanists drink.

However, even though the two primary Chamomiles contain constituents that are not identical, they are similar, related, and similarly used. Chamomile's uses differ little today than from those of 2000 years ago. Those actions include: anti-inflammatory, antiseptic, carminative, antispasmodic, sedative, and wound healing.

The genus name "Matricaria" came from Chamomile's role as a gynecological herb. Historically, it has been used for "nervous diseases and the complaints of women," but the occasional reference to its use for female complaints is not well documented in modern medical literature.

The Egyptians believed in its power to cure ague, a type of malarial fever, and dedicated it to their gods. The Greeks noted its distinct apple scent and named it "ground apple" (*kamai* means on the ground and *melon* an apple), hence its name today, Chamomile. To the Anglo-Saxons, Chamomile was one of nine sacred herbs given to them by the god Woden. The Spanish call it *Manzanillai*, for little apple, and still make a sherry with it.

In the Middle Ages, Chamomile was planted in the walkways of gardens. There is a saying that goes; "Like a Chamomile bed, the more it is trodden, the more it will spread." I tip my hat to something that thrives on being trampled. And, through history, Chamomile has been known as the "plant's physician." Folklore has it that if you have another plant in your garden that is drooping and sickly, place Chamomile near it, and it will recover. If this works, let me know.

While we sip our bedtime Chamomile toddy in the U.S., Europe has taken to Chamomile as something of a cure-all. In fact, the Germans use the phrase *alles zutraut*, which translates to *can do anything*.

Science:
As mentioned above, the constituents are not identical in German and Roman Chamomiles, but similar. They both have volatile oils, flavonoids, Chamazulene, and stuff. Because German chamomile is what we are most likely to be dealing with, we should deal strictly with the phytochemicals in it.

The flower head is the most desirable part of the plant, so much so that medieval herbalists developed double-flowered varieties to increase the yield. They contain a blue-colored volatile oil that contains the principal anti-inflammatory and antispasmodic actives. When extracted, the yield will be between .24-1.9%. The percent of volatile oil present in a commercial preparation may be listed on the label. The key constituents in this oil are alpha-bisabolol, alpha-bisabolol oxides A and B, and matricin, which is converted to chamazulene during the extraction process.

Also among chamomile's active constituents are flavonoids, which include apigenin, luteolin, quercetin, anthemidin, and rutin. While the principle anti-inflammatory and antispasmodic actives come from the volatile oils, we have discovered that flavonoids also possess significant anti-inflammatory activity. This is important as only 10-15% of the volatile oils are retained when chamomile is prepared as a tea from dried plant material.

Chamomile also contains bitter glycosides like anthemic acid, and coumarins like herniarin and umbelliferone, which also exhibit antispasmodic properties. Like most herbal medicines, the therapeutic value of Chamomile does not rest on a single constituent, but on a complex of compounds.

If should be noted that whole extracts of Chamomile preparations with higher concentrations of volatile oils are more effective medicines. Commission E standards require a volatile oil concentration of not less than .4%, but the more the better. Nevertheless, for chronic conditions, teas consumed over long periods of time will accumulate beneficial effects.

Modern Day Uses:

Modern uses of Chamomile are backed not only by centuries of use, but also by intensive recent research. It is very gentle medicine, making it very suitable for children. Even though Americans have relegated Chamomile to a "calming" agent, its most important benefits may be most noteworthy to the gastrointestinal tract. Specifically, Chamomile exerts both anti-inflammatory and antispasmodic activity.

Chamomile could be used for any of the following GI conditions:

> ➢ Cramping or irritation due to stress or diarrhea

> ➤ Indigestion
> ➤ Gastritis
> ➤ Irritable bowel disorders
> ➤ Spastic Colon
> ➤ Crohn's disease
> ➤ Colitis
> ➤ Infant colic
> ➤ Acidity
> ➤ Hiatus hernia
> ➤ Stomach aches
> ➤ Bloating
> ➤ Cramps
> ➤ Flatulence
> ➤ Nausea

Because Chamomile also exerts a mild antimicrobial effect, in addition to being anti-inflammatory and antispasmodic, it should be considered for the following:

> ➤ Peptic ulcers
> ➤ Food poisoning
> ➤ Intestinal Flu

Because of the presence of bitter elements, Chamomile stimulates the production of gastric juices, thus aiding in digestion.

Two side notes worth mentioning are that Chamomile helps prevent ulcer formation induced by alcohol consumption, and, at least in laboratory animals, Chamomile inhibited ulcer formation caused by a nonsteroidal anti-inflammatory drug (NSAID), namely indomethacin, a very strong NSAID, notorious for irritation of the GI tract.

Chamomile's calming effects have been validated. Apigenin, one of its predominant flavonoids, was shown to have a clear anxiolytic activity. It actually has an affinity to the same receptor sites that benzodiazepine (Valium®) drugs do. Commercial preparations may begin listing the percent of Apigenin present in their plant extract, with 1-1.5% better ensuring effectiveness.

On the stress front, Chamomile can be used for:

> ➢ Mild sleep disorders (especially in children)
> ➢ Nightmares in children
> ➢ Hyperactivity in children
> ➢ Restlessness
> ➢ Teething
> ➢ General stress
> ➢ Anxiety
> ➢ Menstrual cramps

Topically, Chamomile also has anti-inflammatory properties in addition to promoting wound healing and antibacterial activities. Typical uses might include:

> ➢ Inflammatory skin conditions like eczema, insect bites, poison oak, and bed sores
> ➢ General wound healing
> ➢ Mouthwash for canker sores and mouth and gum irritations
> ➢ Hemorrhoids
> ➢ Hair tint and conditioner
> ➢ Diaper rash
> ➢ Bacterial skin diseases

Another interesting application of Chamomile is that it can be used as an inhalant for inflammations and irritations of the respiratory tract. Consider trying Chamomile in a vaporizer or humidifier for chronic obstructive pulmonary disorders and asthma.

Dose:

For topical use, a compress works well, unless a commercially manufactured cream or ointment is more appropriate, practical, or convenient. One way to apply a compress is to first make tea. Then saturate cotton cloth with the tea and wrap it on the affected area. Now, wrap around the cloth with plastic wrap. If you like, you can apply alternating hot and cold on top of the cloth. Apply heat for twelve minutes, then ice for four minutes. Do this for at least one hour, two to three times daily.

Tea is made by steeping ½ teaspoonful to a tablespoonful of dried
flowers in very warm water for 5-10 minutes. Cover the container so
as to not lose too much of the volatile oils. Pass your tea through a
strainer and have a cup 3-4 times daily. Or if you're as lazy as I am,
open 4-6 capsules and make your tea. Actually, I am so lazy that I
would probably swallow the capsules, drink the water, jump up and
down, and let the tea be made in my stomach.

The truth is that I would probably also use an "extract," which is more
concentrated. I would only have to take one 500 mg high volatile oil/
Apigenin capsule, 3-4 times daily. Or, if I wanted to have a tea, I
would use a tincture that was concentrated to around a 4:1 or 5:1, and
add the appropriate number of drops to very warm (no steam) water.

For children, the general rule of thumb is to give one-half the adult
dose, unless the product is already formulated for children. Then,
follow the label instructions.

Cautions:

There are scanty and poorly supported references to Chamomile's use
as an emmenagogue, an agent which could stimulate menses. This
would preclude its use in pregnancy. However, our most respected
resources recommend its use for morning sickness. In fact, European
monographs, including Commission E, list no contraindications to the
use of chamomile during pregnancy and lactation, and no interactions
with commonly prescribed medicines. It should also be noted that the
references to Chamomile's uterine stimulation seem to be for Roman
Chamomile, and for whole plant and not the flowers. However, if one
wanted to be overly cautious, avoid large doses of Chamomile in the
1st trimester of pregnancy, and use only the German variety.

Side effects are rare with Chamomile used internally. Allergic reactions are possible but don't happen often. In fact, within about a
hundred-year window, ending in 1982, only 50 reports of allergies
were documented. And of the 50, only five were attributed to German
Chamomile.

Chamomile is a member of the daisy family. So, if you are allergic to
ragweed, asters, or chrysanthemums, and you don't want to be case

number six, proceed with care. Roman Chamomile is much more likely to cause a skin reaction in an allergic person.

References:

See General Resources

Schilcher, H and Hansel, H. *Lehrbuch der Pharmakognosie und Phytopharmazie*, 4th Ed. Springer-Verlag. Berlin, 1988

Farnsworth, N and Morgan, B. *Journal of the American Medical Association* 221:410, 1972

Grieve, M. *A Modern Herbal*. New York, NY. Dover Publications. 1971

Habersang, S, et al. "Pharmacological Studies with Compounds of Chamomile. Studies on Toxicity of Alpha Bisabolol." *Planta Medica*. 1979; 37:115

Hamon, N. "Herbal Medicine. The Chamomiles." *Can Pharm J.* 1989; Nov:612

O'Hara, M, et al. "A Review of 12 Commonly Used Medicinal Herbs." *Arch Fam Med.* 1998; 7:523-536

Tyler, V. *Herbs of Choice*. New York, Hawthorn Press Inc. 1994

Viola, H, et al. "Apigenin, a Component of Matricaria recutita Flowers, is a Central Benzodiazepine Receptor-Ligand with Anxiolytic Effects." *Planta Med.* 1995; 61:213-6

Matricaria flos. ESCOP Monograph,

Mann, C, Staba E. "The Chemistry, Pharmacology, and Commercial Formulations of Chamomile." *Herbs, Spices, and Medicinal Plants: Recent Advances in Botany, Horticulture, and Pharmacology*. Phoenix, AZ. Oryx Press. 1986

Chaste Tree

(Vitex agnus-castus)

Other Common Names:
Chasteberry, Monk's Pepper, Monk's Pepper Tree, Abraham's Balm, Chase Lamb Tree, Safe Tree, Gatillier, Hemp Tree, Keuschbaum

Background:
Vitex is a small shrub native to Greece and Italy; however, it is now naturalized to warm climates in the Untied States, Asia, and Europe. Its peppery dried fruit has been used medicinally for thousands of years.

Vitex has two historic stories to tell. One is based on old wives tales and has no scientific foundation. The other shows the amazing insight of early healers whose writings are being validated by modern science over 2000 years later.

The fairy tale is that Vitex has a history of being used as an anti-aphrodisiac. In ancient Rome, vestal virgins carried twigs of Vitex as a symbol of their chastity. The Greeks would spread berries in the beds of their soldier's wives to assure that they would remain faithful while they were away at war. In Italy during the Middle Ages, flowers were scattered along the walkways leading to convents and monasteries as recruits passed by. Moreover, Vitex blossoms were spread around monasteries to deter monks from running off into town and monkeying around. Not to mention that they fed them the ground dried berries as a spice, hence the name monk's pepper.

Needless to say, if these tactics worked, it was for some other reason. Scientifically speaking, if Vitex increases luteinizing hormone, which it appears to, this would actually favor the balance of hormones towards testosterone, thus increasing libido, not quelling it. That would go for both men and women.

The name is even derived from this nonsense. The species name Agnus castus originates from the Latin *castitas*, meaning chastity, as does the English name Chaste Tree.

On the other hand, I am amazed at how "right on" the ancients were with Vitex. Hippocrates, in the 4th century BC, prescribed Vitex for hemorrhaging following childbirth and for assisting the passing of childbirth. The Roman healer Pliny (23-79 AD) wrote about Vitex as trees that furnish menstruation. And 200 years ago, American physicians were prescribing Vitex to increase milk production and menstrual disorders, just like today.

Science:

The exact actives of Vitex are unknown. However, there are unique compounds to which the plant is generally standardized. They include the glycosides agnuside, aucubin, and eurostosid.

Pharmacologically, Vitex has a corpus luteum action on the body. That is, it seems to increase luteinizing hormone (LH) while inhibiting the release of follicle stimulating hormone (FSH). The net result is a shift in the estrogen-progesterone ratio in the direction of progesterone. It also contains an active ingredient or combination of ingredients that binds to dopamine receptor sites in the pituitary, inhibiting prolactin release. While Vitex inhibits prolactin secretion, recent research has confused us about its progesterogneic mechanisms.

Modern Day Uses:

> Abnormal menstrual rhythm
> Excessively prolonged menses
> Profuse menses
> Scanty menstruation
> Abnormally heavy menstruation
> Abnormally long menstruation
> Absence of menstruation
> Painful menstruation
> Suppressed menstruation
> Breast pain
> Premenstrual acne
> PMS
> Premenstrual lip herpes
> Infertility

> ➢ Endometriosis
> ➢ Menopause
> ➢ Peri-menopause
> ➢ Increase milk production
> ➢ Uterine bleeding

Dose:

Vitex is generally dosed once daily, in the morning. Take per manufacturer's directions for standardized extracts. For non-standardized capsules, take up to 2 gm daily.

Vitex is not a fast-acting herb. You must be patient with it. It may take four to six months to do its job. In the case of infertility, it may even take up to 18 months.

Cautions:

There have not been significant side effects associated with Vitex. In one market survey, only 17 of 1542 women discontinued use due to untoward events. Keeping in mind that nearly all of these women had hormone imbalances, the percentage becomes almost insignificant. The most common problems were dermatological in nature.

When used for milk production, chemically analyzed breast milk showed no compositional changes after Vitex administration. That means it is safe to use even while breast feeding.

References:

See General Resources

Brown, D. "Vitex Agnus Castus: Clinical Monograph." *Quarterly Review of Natural Medicine*. Summer 1994

Ditmar, F, et al. "Premenstrual Syndrome: Treatment with a Phytopharmaceutical." *Therpiewoche Gynakol*. 1992; 5:60-8

Gerhard, I, et al. "Mastodynon® for Female Infertility. Randomized, Placebo Controlled, Clinical Double-Blind Study." *Res in Comp Med*. 1998; 5:272-8

Houghton, P. "Agnus Castus." *Pharm J*. 1994; 253:720-1

Lauritien, C, et al. "Treatment of Premenstrual Syndrome with Vitex Agnus Castus.

Controlled, Double-Blind Study Versus Pyridoxine." *Phytomedicine*. 1997. 4:183-189

Leonhardt, J, et al. "*In Vitro* Prolactin but not LH and FSH Release is Inhibited by Compounds in Extracts of Agnus Castus: Direct Evidence for a Dopaminergic Principle by the Dopamine Receptor Assay." *Exp Clin Endocrinol*. 1994; 102:448-454

Loch, E, et al. "The Treatment of Menstrual disorders with Vitex Agnus-Castus Tincture." *Der Frauemarzt*. 1991; 32:867-70

Milewicz, A, et al. "Vitex Agnus-Castus Extract in the Treatment of Luteal Phase Defects Due to Latent Hyperprolactinemia: Results of a Randomized Placebo-Controlled Double-Blind Study." *Arzneim Forsch Drug Res*. 1993; 43:752-6

Peteres-Welter, C, et al. "Menstrual Abnormalities and PMS. Vitex Agnus-Castus in a Study of Application." *Therapiewoche Gynakol*. 1994; 7:49-52

Propping, D, et al. "Diagnosis and Therapy of Corpus Luteum Deficiency in General Practice." *Therapiewoche*. 1988; 38:2992-3001

Snow, J. "Vitex Agnus-Castus L." *The Protocol Journal of Botanical Medicine*. 1996; Spring:20-23

Turner, S, et al. "A Double-Blind Clinical Trial on a Herbal Remedy for PMS; a Case Study." *Comp Ther Med*. 1993; 1:73-7

Cranberry

(Vaccinium macrocarpon)

Other Common Names:
Marsh Wort, Fenne Berry

Background:
The original name of Cranberry was actually Craneberry. It was named for the fruit's bird-shaped blossom. The word first appeared in a letter written by a Cape Cod missionary named John Eliot in 1647. Native Americans thought that Cranberries were a gift from the Great Spirit, having been dropped from the beak of a dove into the swamps. They used the red berries to dye blankets and make pemmican, a food made of crushed berries, fat, and dried meat. It was also used as a medicine to extract poison from wounds.

The Indians called the berry *Ibimi* when they introduced it to the Pilgrims. They, in turn, found that after sweetening the berries, they made an excellent sauce for meats. They made the Cranberry sauce we are familiar with today, in addition to tarts, jams and syrups.

As young America's trade grew with Europe, Cranberries were loaded onto sailing ships to supplement the crew's vitamin C, hence preventing scurvy. Other 17th century uses of Cranberry included liver and gallbladder disorders, gastric ailments, blood problems, and even cancer.

Science:
Key constituents of Cranberry center around its organic acids and polyphenols. The polyphenols include proanthocyanins and anthocyanins and are responsible for its antioxidant activity. Its organic acids include hippuric acid, ellagic acid, and quinic acid, and may be the actives directly related to Cranberry's effect on the urinary system. Cranberry extracts are usually standardized on the quinic acid.

The primary focus on which Cranberry has claimed its fame, other than as a Thanksgiving condiment, is its effect on the urinary tract.

Since the turn of the century, Cranberry has been thought to be beneficial in reducing bladder infections. In a 1914 study, researchers reported that Cranberries were high in benzoic acid, and that when it was excreted in the urine, it was excreted as hippuric acid. The theory from that time through the 1970s was that acidification of the urine was the mechanism through which Cranberry worked.

However, because the concentration of hippuric acid in the urine is insufficient to inhibit bacteria, another explanation was sought. Recent studies have shown Cranberry to significantly reduce the ability of bacteria to adhere to the lining of the bladder and urethra. Therefore, the likelihood of infection is greatly reduced as bacteria must first adhere to the mucosal lining before they can set up housekeeping.

Only juices of the Vaccinium genus have this effect. Cranberry and blueberry have specifically been tested, but Bilberry and Bearberry (Uva-Ursi) are also members of this family. Uva-Ursi has been used extensively as a urinary diuretic and antiseptic. Perhaps Uva-Ursi also has this secondary effect.

An interesting side note on Cranberry juice is that it also has the ability to selectively inhibit the adhesion of plaque building bacteria in the mouth. Currently, the main methods for decreasing dental plaque are brushing and flossing. Perhaps one day, we will be washing our mouths out with a Cranberry mouthwash. The only draw back is that real Cranberry juice is almost too tart to tolerate. On the other hand, Cranberry cocktail contains about 12% sugar, which is known to promote plaque aggregation and dental cavities. It seems that researchers still have a little work to do in this area.

Modern Day Uses:

Urinary tract infections result in upwards of 5 million physician office visits annually. Cranberry can help mitigate the symptoms and frequency of these infections, suffered by millions of Americans, mostly women. I believe this makes Cranberry one of the many supplements that can make an impact in curbing healthcare dollars needlessly spent. I especially advocate the use of Cranberry for non-pregnant, sexually active women with a history of recurrent urinary tract infections.

Many individuals have resorted to drinking large quantities of Cranberry juice. I am not a great advocate of drinking Cranberry juice. Most juices are watered down and contain sugar. In addition to not being beneficial to the immune system, sugar is a source of empty wasted calories. An 8 oz. serving of juice could cost a weight watcher an additional 140 calories.

Cranberry extracts are available in concentrated tablet or capsule form, some as concentrated as 34:1. That is, it takes 34 pounds of Cranberry to make 1 pound of extract. Additionally, better extracts will contain ellagic acid, a phytochemical that shows promise as a chemoprotective. Cranberry juice does not contain this acid.

Cranberry supplements could be considered for any of the following urinary problems:

> Frequency
> Urgency/Leakage
> Burning
> Pain/Stinging
> Straining
> Voiding in small amounts

Dose:
If you can find one of the new concentrated extracts, like the 34:1 mentioned above, a once daily dose of 500mg. is all you need as a preventative. More heroic efforts, including other complementary herbs, may be required for acute infections.

Cautions:
None known.

References:
See General Resources

Avorn, J. et al. "Reduction of Bacteriuria and Pyuria after Ingestion of Cranberry Juice." *JAMA*. 1994; 271:751-4

Bodel, R. et al. "Cranberry Juice and the Antibacterial Action of Hippuric Acid." *J Lab Clin Med* 1959; 54:881

Gibson et al. *Journal of Naturpathic Medicine.* 1991; 2:45-47 (Missing name of article) Will check it out.

Sobota, A. "Inhibition of Bacterial Adherence by Cranberry Juice: Potential Use for the Treatment of Urinary Tract Infections." *Journal of Urology.* 1984; 131:1013

Schmidt, D., Sobata, A. "An Examination of the Anti-Adherence Activity of Cranberry Juice on Urinary and Non-Urinary Isolates." *Micorbios.* 1988; 55:173

Sternlieb, P. "Cranberry Juice in Renal Disease." *New Eng J Med.* 1963; 268:57

Walker, E. et al. "Cranberry Concentrate: UTI Prophylaxis." *J Family Pact.* 1997; 45:167-8

Weiss, E. et al. "Inhibiting Interspecies Coaggregation of Plaque Bacteria with a Cranberry Juice Constituent." *Journal of the American Dental Association.* 1998; 129:1719-23

Zafriri, D. et al. "Inhibitory Activity of Cranberry Juice on Adherence of Type I and Type II Fimbriated E Coli to Eucaryotic Cells." *Antimicro Agents Chem.* 1989; 33:92

Damiana

(Turnera aphrodisiaca)

Other Common Names:
Herba de la Pastora, Mexican Damiana, Old Woman's Broom

Background:
Damiana, if to say nothing else, is controversial. Some medical folks and sex therapists praise it; some consider it a hoax, and some are undecided. I personally couldn't pass up the opportunity to look a little deeper into a botanical that had aphrodisiac as part of its name.

Damiana is a scraggly shrub native to tropical Mexico, but it can also be found in western Central America and the West Indies. It has been used to treat colic, bed-wetting, menstrual and menopausal problems, water retention, depression, anxiety, and bronchial problems, and it has a long-standing reputation as an aphrodisiac. The leaves of the plant have been traditionally used to treat frigidity in women and impotence in men. Damiana has also been associated with inducing erotic dreams when taken at bedtime.

According to folk history, Damiana has been used for centuries by Mexican women, who traditionally drink a cup of tea made from the leaves an hour of so before having sex. In the 1870s, an American pharmaceutical firm, Helmick and Company, introduced the plant as a powerful aphrodisiac to improve the sexual ability of the enfeebled and aged. An elixir and extract of Damiana was listed as an official drug in the *National Formulary* from 1888 to 1916, and the extract stayed in it until 1947.

Science:
I was not able to find any reasonable evidence in the scientific literature to confirm Damiana's aphrodisiac qualities. However, reputable Herbalists like David Hoffman, author of the *Herbalist* and *An Elder's Herbal* considers Damiana to have definite action on the central nervous system as well as the hormonal system.

The leaves contain .2 to .9% volatile oil, 14% resin, about 3.5% tannin, 6% starch, and a bitter substance called daminanian. The oil's alkaloids may increase circulation and are believed to have a direct, mildly irritating, effect on the urinary tract. This enhanced circulation and mild irritation, like a mild peristalsis, may subsequently account for the aphrodisiac effect that has eluded modern science.

Modern Day Uses:

Damiana is considered by Chinese traditions as a *Yang* tonic. That is, a tonic that strengthens the energy and vitality of the body, including the sexual energy. I am more likely to trust the wisdom of the Chinese and their *Yin Yangs* (no pun intended), than I am the judgment of someone selling sex aids in the Wild West off of a medicine show wagon. Additionally, I believe that where there is smoke, there is fire. Spanish missionaries reported that the Mexican Indians prepared a drink of Damiana leaves and drank it for its love-enhancing properties. One has to respect the notion that Indian customs are customs for a reason. Therefore, I will come down on the side of the undecided. There are no significant side effects associated with Damiana, so if you are so inclined, go for it.

Damiana is not usually used alone, but in combination with other similar or complementary herbs. It is used in the Caribbean, by boiling the leaves and inhaling the vapors to relieve headaches. Damiana teas are also said to aid in the control of bedwetting.

Dose:

Follow label instructions.

Cautions:

None known.

References:

See General Resources

Duke, J. *The Green Pharmacy*. Emmaus, PA, Rodale Press. 1997

Miller, R. *The Magical and Ritual Use of Aphrodisiacs*. New York, NY. Destiny Books. 1985

Lininger, S. et al. *The Natural Pharmacy*. Rocklin, CA. Prima Publishing. 1998

Pedersen, M. *Nutritional Herbology*. Warsaw, IN. Wendell W. Whitman Co. 1995

Watson, C. *Love Potions: A Guide to Aphrodisiacs and Sexual Pleasures*. Los Angeles, CA. Tarcher. 1993

Dandelion

(Taraxacum officinale)

Other Common Names:
Lion's tooth, Priest's Crown, Wild Endive, Fairy Clock, Swine's Snout, Blowball, Milk Gowan, White Endive, Cankerwort, Irish Daisy

Background:
Dandelion was used by Arab physicians as far back as the 10th century. It is likely that its genus name Taraxacum is derived from the Arabic word for edible *tharakcharkon*, but equally likely that it came from the Geek, *taraxo* for ailment, and *akos* for pain.

Food, drug, or both
Historically, Dandelion's leaves were probably more known as an early spring salad, and its root material as a substitute for coffee. Dandelion is not only a wonderful plant medicine but has, and continues to be consumed as a nutritious food and beverage. The leaves, in addition to making a fine salad, can be cooked like spinach. And, the plant is related to chicory, which explains how it came to be a coffee substitute, albeit without the stimulant properties.

Yummy tidings aside, Dandelion has long been used in herbal remedies for diabetes and disorders of the liver, in addition to being used as a laxative, tonic, appetite stimulant, digestant, and stimulant of bile flow. The great English botanist/surgeon/barber, John Gerard (1545-1612), described its mechanism of action as it, "doth withall clense and open by reason of the bitterness."

Wee wee or a tooth
But of the multitude of uses for which Dandelion was acclaimed, its employment for kidney and urinary problems was best known, and certainly most colorful. The common name Dandelion comes for the French, *dent de lion*, referring to the plant's lion's tooth leaves. However, the French are more likely to refer to the plant as *piss au lit*, which translates to "wet the bed," referring to its strong diuretic action. "Wet the bed" might be a better name, because, quite honestly, I have

never been able to see the similarity of a Dandelion leaf to a lion's tooth.

When the plant has seeded and the florets close up, some say it resembles the snout of a pig (Swine's Snout). When all the seeds have flown and the flower disc is bare, it was said to resemble the bare head of medieval priests (Priest's Crown); and in old England, children used to play a game to see how many puffs it would take to disperse the seeds (Blowball); and sometimes this game was used to guess the time (Fairy Clock).

Dandelion was not mentioned in Chinese herbal medicine until the 7th century. Unlike Western herbal medicine, which divides the leaf and root, the Chinese use the whole plant, which they call *Pu Gong Ying*. Today in China, Dandelion is used to treat breast problems including cancer, mastitis, and lactation problems. In modern Europe, it is used to treat fever and various skin problems that benefit from detoxification, as well as the typical liver and digestive ailments.

Science:

Dandelion contains an abundance of terpenoid and sterol bitters (principally taraxacin and taraxacerin). Like Gerard suggested in his day, these bitter principals are responsible for its primary therapeutic actions. It also contains a large amount of polysaccharides (primarily fructosans and inulin).

Hepatic effects

Bitters aid digestion by stimulating the secretion of digestive agents. They begin by increasing salivation, invigorating gastric juices, and end by stimulating the release of bile by the liver and gallbladder.

Dandelion's actions are twofold. First, it acts on the liver to increase bile production and flow to the gallbladder. This effect is called a choleretic effect. Second, it works on the gallbladder to initiate greater contractions and hence release of stored bile. This effect is called a cholagogue effect.

Glucose effect

Dandelion seems to have sugar regulating activity. This is probably, at least in part, due to its high inulin content. Inulin is a polysaccharide fiber, made up of repeating fructose sugar molecules. The presence of inulin is thought to prevent vacillations in blood sugar levels. It is this stabilization that may contribute to Dandelion's alleged weight loss benefits, as unstable blood sugar levels tend to lead to erratic eating patterns.

Diuretic effect

Dandelion leaves have long been used as a diuretic. In one study on mice, dandelion was shown to have activity comparable to the pharmaceutical furosemide. This could prove to be valuable to those with pet mice facing congestive heart failure effects. But regardless of whether Dandelion's diuretic effects are of interest to you or your pet mouse, you will be pleased to know that the plant is high in potassium, a mineral that generally needs replacing with diuresis, making it self-correcting.

Cancer effect

Animal models have demonstrated Dandelion's ability to inhibit the growth of cancer cells. Japanese researchers in 1981 isolated a glucose polymer from the plant that had anti-tumor properties. This lends credence to the Chinese use of Dandelion for breast cancer.

Modern Day Uses:

Dandelion is actually three different botanical medicines. Dandelion leaf extract is used primarily for its diuretic effects, and Dandelion root is used primarily for its effects on the liver. And, if you let the flower go to seed, to blow the seeds off the Dandelion is to send one's thoughts to a loved one. So, Dandelion technically even has an effect on the heart.

Leaf preparations - diuretic, digestive tonic (as a tea)
Root preparations - Liver tonic, promotes bile flow, cholecystitis, gallstones, jaundice, mild laxative, antirheumatic.

Night blindness and weed control

Almost all the fuss made about Dandelion goes to its leaves and roots.

Well, the flowers may prove to offer up a benefit one day. Nicholas Culpeper, the revolutionary in medicine of the mid 1600s, was once overheard saying (I guess), "This herb helps one to see farther without a pair of spectacles." According to data presented in the *Journal of the American Medical Association*, the flowers contain a substance called helenin. This substance appears to enhance vision for those who may have a problem with night vision. Now, for those who want to try to improve their night vision, while simultaneously ridding their yard of pesky Dandelion garden volunteers, try making Dandelion wine.

All you need is:

> ➢ 1 gallon of unsprayed Dandelion flowers
> ➢ pure boiling water
> ➢ 3 oranges
> ➢ 3 lemons
> ➢ 5 ½ cups natural brown sugar
> ➢ yeast

Directions:

1. Wash about a gallon's worth of dandelion flowers thoroughly in cold water, pull off stalks and other green parts, and place in a large plastic pail.

2. Finely chop the colored outer rind of three oranges and three lemons, add to flowers, then cover with boiling water. Cover pail with plastic or cloth, and let sit for three days, stirring twice daily.

3. After three days, strain the juice into a large kettle, squeezing or pressing to extract as much liquid as possible. Add about 5 1/2 cups natural brown sugar, and cook juice at a medium boil for about 30 minutes. Let cool to room temperature (around 70 degrees), and then mix in wine making yeast (as recommended by a wine making supply store professional or the package label).

4. Divide the mixture between two clean gallon jugs and seal tops with fermentation locks (also found at winemaking supply stores).

5. When fermentation slows (one to three days), siphon all the liquid into one bottle, filling it to 1 inch below the stopper. Add one tablespoon of strong tea. Then reseal with fermentation lock and let ferment at warm room temperature until the bubbling stops (one to four weeks).

6. Siphon as often as necessary to clear wine, adding enough liquid each time to fill bottle to 1 inch from stopper. When wine is clear, bottle, cork, and label "Night Blindness Medicine."

Dose:

Dandelion is one of those herbs that we kind of use the way "The Maker" has prepared it. It is not standardized to an active, only concentrated, perhaps to a 4:1 extract. Take 500mg three times daily, or as directed by a health care professional.

Cautions:

Dandelion is non-toxic, and no documented side effects have been reported. Occasionally, contact with the fresh leaves or the milky latex may cause an allergic reaction in sensitive individuals.

According to the German Federal Institute of Pharmaceutical and Medicinal Products, the treatment of gallstones with Dandelion should be done with medical supervision. If bile ducts are obstructed, Dandelion should not be used at all.

Since Dandelion may have mild anti-diabetic and blood pressure reducing actions, it is advisable to monitor these respective conditions more closely if you are going to use the herb. It is always a good idea to let your physician be a participant in your complementary treatments.

Similarly, if you are taking diuretic medication, taking Dandelion leaf preparations may potentate your medication and adversely effect your electrolyte balance. The concomitant use is not advisable.

References:

See General Resources

Aesoph, L. "Herbs & Nutrients for Weight Loss." *Delicious*. 1996; January:46-49

Akhtar, M. et al. "Effects of Portulaca oleracae and Taraxacum Officinale in Normoglycemic and Alloxan-Treated Hyperglycemic Rabbits." *J Pak Med Assoc*. 1985; 35:207-210

ESCOP, *Monographs on the Medicinal Use of Plant Drugs*. Exeter, England. ESCOP Secretariat. 1997

Grieve, M. *A Modern Herbal*. New York, NY. Dover Publications. 1971

http://www.noahsays.com/cooking/17.htm

Lust, J. *The Herb Book*. New York, NY. Bantam Books. 1983

Racz-Kotilla E. et al. "The Action of Taraxacum Officinale Extracts on the Body Weight and Diuresis of Laboratory Animals." *Planta Med*. 1974; 26:212-217

Tierra, M. *The Way of Herbs*. New York, NY. Pocket Books. 1990

Wagner, H. & Wolff, P. eds. *New Natural Products and Plant Drugs with Pharmacological, Biological or Therapeutic Activity*. Heidelberg, Germany. Springer-Verlag. 1977

Devil's Claw

(Harpagophytum procumbens)

Other Common Names:
Grapple Plant, Wood Spider

Background:
Devil's Claw is a shrubby vine native to southwest Africa, namely the Kalahari Desert, Namibian Steppes, and the island of Madagascar. Its name makes reference to claw-shaped mini grappling hooks that wrap around the plant's seeds. These hooks serve to disperse the seeds by sticking to a passing animal. The plant has nothing to do with Satan, instead getting its name from the translation of the German name *Heufelskralle*. This is all well and interesting, except that it is the root that is the source of Devil's Claw's actives.

The root, actually underground tubers, is highly valued by indigenous African Bushmen, Hottentots, and Bantu as a bitter tonic for digestion, and also for arthritic conditions. They have also used it for fever, as a blood purifier, and to ease the pain of potentially painful childbirths. Externally, it was used for boils and various other sores.

Europeans traveling to Africa became interested in the health benefits of Devil's Claw and brought some back home for testing. Since 1958, Devil's Claw has found its way into European herbal medicine based on generally favorable test results.

Science:
The principal active ingredient to which the properties of Devil's Claw are attributed is harpagoside, an iridoid glucoside. The secondary tubers of the plant contain twice as much harpagoside as the primary root. While it is believed that other components are involved in Devil Claw's analgesic and anti-inflammatory actions, medicinal preparations are nonetheless standardized to harpagoside in concentrations ranging from .1 to 5%.

While not by the same mechanisms by which standard pharmaceutical drugs exert their anti-inflammatory activity (alteration of arachidonic acid metabolism-for the one person reading this who was wondering), animal and human studies show harpagoside to possess the same anti-inflammatory effects. One German study indicated that Devil's Claw anti-inflammatory activity was comparable to the pharmaceutical, phenylbutazone.

Extracts of Devil's Claw have, in animal models, been shown to affect smooth muscles due to a complex interaction of its constituents on cholinergic receptors. They caused a dose related reduction in blood pressure, decreased heart rate, and exerted a protective effect with regard to arrhythmias (irregular heart beats).

Modern Day Uses:
In Europe, modern uses include the following:

> ➢ Appetite stimulant
> ➢ Digestive aide
> ➢ Analgesic
> ➢ Anti-inflammatory
> ➢ Tendonitis
> ➢ Supportive therapy of degenerative diseases of the extremities
> ➢ Acute low back pain

Dose:
As an anti-inflammatory/analgesic agent, use a standardized extract, and take the equivalent of about 50mg harpagoside daily. For example, if a preparation is standardized to 3% harpagoside, then each 100mg of extract yields 3mg harpagoside. If you can find 555mg capsules, take 1 capsule three times daily. If you can't find a capsule like this, come as close as you can. This becomes less of an issue when one considers that many times Devil's Claw is synergistically combined with complementary herbs.

The European Scientific Cooperative on Phytotherapy recommends that the duration of treatment for arthritic use should be two to three months. So, be patient.

For other uses of Devil's Claw, follow label directions.

Cautions:

The German Federal Institute of Pharmaceutical and Medicinal Products lists no known side effects or interactions with other drugs. However, I would like to offer a few words of wisdom with which to come down on the side of caution.

One of the ways Devil's Claw may improve digestion is via its promoting the secretion of stomach acid. Therefore, it should probably not be used by persons suffering from ulcers. This may be a non-issue when the plant is used in combination mixtures, but nonetheless, be aware.

Secondly, since Devil's Claw can positively affect heart rhythm, one cannot discount the possibility that it may have some effect on the actions of other antiarrhythmics. Pay attention.

References:

See General Resources

Baghdikian, B, et al. "An Analytical Study, Anti-inflammatory and Analgesic Effects of Harpagophytum procumbens and Harpagophytum zeyheri." *Planta Med.* 1997; 63:171-76

Chrubasik, S. et al. "Effectiveness of Harpagophytum Procumbens in Treatment of Acute Low Back Pain." *Phytomedicine.* 1996; 3:1-10

DerMarderosian, A ed. *Review of Natural Products.* St. Louis, MO, Facts and Comparisons, 1999

ESCOP, *Monographs on the Medicinal Use of Plant Drugs.* Exeter, England. ESCOP Secretariat. 1997

Lininger, S. et al. *The Natural Pharmacy.* Rocklin, CA. Prima Publishing. 1998

Pedersen, M. *Nutritional Herbology.* Warsaw, IN. Wendell W. Whitman Co. 1995

Dong Quai

(Angelica sinensis)

Other Common Names:
Tang Kuei, Dang Qui, Chinese Angelica, Dry Kuei, Women's Ginseng

Background:
Dong Quai is an ancient Traditional Chinese Medicine (TCM) that is classified as a tonifying herb. Tonifying herbs are those that strengthen or supplement an area or process of the body that is out of balance. Tonic herbs strengthen the body's defenses against disease but are not to be used when one is acutely ill. TCM practitioners will correct any acute ailments before using a tonic. If you become ill, they will discontinue using any tonic you may be on. In the spirit of TCM belief, the meridians that Dong Quai supports are the heart, liver, spleen and kidney. Dong Quai means "proper order," and it is used to return body systems to just that.

Dong Quai is native to China where it has a reputation perhaps second only to Ginseng. For thousands of years, it has been cultivated for medicinal use, and particularly for female disorders. As primarily a women's remedy, Dong Quai has been and is today used for such conditions as dysmenorrhea and amenorrhea (difficulty with and absence of menses), and menopause symptoms. It has also been used for other conditions including abdominal pain, blood disorders, rheumatism, migraines, ulcers, constipation, high blood pressure and convalescence.

Science:
The part of the plant used for medicine is the root. About six coumarin derivatives have been isolated that exhibit vasodilatory, antispasmodic, and central nervous system stimulant properties. Working backwards, this may explain, in part, mechanisms for some of the traditional uses. Scientific investigation has also uncovered components of essential oils and flavonoids that may explain Dong Quai's purported hormonal, analgesic, and immuno-modulating activity.

The hormonal actions of Dong Quai do not seem to come from estrogenic activity. It appears to act more by increasing blood flow and reducing vascular resistance. It also has confirmed anti-inflammatory activity coupled with its ability to reduce spasms and pain.

Modern Day Uses:

In China, Dong Quai is a frequently prescribed medicine, generally combined with other herbs. It is used to support and maintain normal reproductive function, lessen pelvic congestion and stop pain caused by congealed blood, such as bruises, menstrual clots and even uterine fibroids. In the West, it is commonly used for:

> ➢ Menstrual difficulties
> ➢ PMS
> ➢ Menopausal difficulties

Dose:

Dong Quai is often standardized to a marker in its essential oil called ligustilide to ensure consistency. Look for about 1% ligustilide, and take 200mg three times daily, unless otherwise directed by the manufacture's or a practitioner's recommendations.

Cautions:

Pregnant and nursing women should use Dong Quai only under the care of a qualified practitioner of Tradition Chinese Medicine.In some people who are hypersensitive to this herb, occasional fever or excessive bleeding may occur. In TCM, Dong Quai is used as a laxative and may therefore cause or exacerbate loose bowels in some people.

References:

Duke, J. *The Green Pharmacy*. Emmaus, PA, Rodale Press. 1997

Huang, K. *The Pharmacology of Chinese Herbs*. Boca Raton, FL. CRC Press. 1993

Noe, J. "Angelica Sinensis: A Monograph." *Journal of Naturopathic Medicine*. 1997; Winter:66-72

Traditional Chinese Medicine and Pharmacology. CD Ver. 1.0. Hopkins, MN. Hopkins Technology. 1995

Echinacea

(Echinacea angustifollia; E. purpurea; E. pallida)

Other Common Names:

American Cone Flower, Black Sampson Root, Black Susans, Brauneria, Cock Up Hat, Comb Flower, Hedgehog, Indian Head, Kansas Snakeroot, Missouri Snakeroot, Narrow-Leaved Purple Cone-flower, Purple Coneflower, Red Sunflower, Rudbeckia, Scurvy Root Snakeroot

Background:

Echinacea is one of the most, if not the most, used and recognizable medicinal plant in the United States today. It is a native American plant, indigenous to the prairie states like Kansas, Missouri, and Nebraska, but ranges from Saskatchewan in the North, to Texas in the South. There are -nine species of Echinacea, with purpurea, angustifollia, and pallida being the primary medical varieties. The name Echinacea comes from the Greek work *echinos*, meaning hedge-hog or sea urchin, a reference to the thorny scales of the dried seed.

From Native Americans to the Eclectics

Echinacea was a gift to Western medicine by the Native American Peoples. It is one of the most important medicinals they shared with European settlers. This versatile plant was used by the Cheyenne, Chocktaw, Comanche, Crow, Dakota, Delaware, Lakota, Omaha, Pawnee, and Winnebago. They used it for sores of the mouth, gums and throat, toothaches, coughs, colds, tonsillitis, sepsis, gonorrhea, colic, bowel inflammation, cramps, anesthesia, and as an eyewash.

The first written mention of Echinacea in medicine appears in L.T. Gronovius' *Flora Virginica* in 1762. Based on notes of an English botanist, John Clayton, who lived in Virginia for 40 years, Echinacea was praised as being valuable for treating the saddle sores of horses.

The first commercial product containing Echinacea was introduced in the U.S. around 1870 by H.C.F. Meyer, a lay doctor from Nebraska, who claimed it as a wonder cure and called it *Meyer's Blood Purifier*.

He learned about Echinacea from the Indians, used it for almost every conceivable malady, and actually achieved many positive outcomes, specifically with snakebites and infections. Meyer is credited with bringing Echinacea to the attention of Eclectic physician Dr. John King, and John Uri Lloyd of Lloyd Brothers Pharmacists, Inc, of Cincinnati, Ohio. Meyer was so convinced of the efficacy of his blood purifier that he offered to travel to Cincinnati and be bitten by a rattle-snake to prove the value of his secret formula. King and Lloyd didn't go for it, but Echinacea was on its way.

Dr. King was instrumental in introducing the use of Echinacea to his medical colleagues. Early Eclectic uses were based on early Native uses. It was used for boils, carbuncles, abscesses, inflammation of lymph glands, and blood poisoning. They also used it for syphilis, gonorrhea, and skin disorders like eczema, psoriasis, acne and poison ivy.

The Eclectics primarily used E. angustifollia. In the 1920s, a German doctor, interested in cultivating this species for the purpose of conduct-ing scientific research, imported seeds. What he ended up getting was seeds of E. purpurea, and thus the next 70 years of medical research on Echinacea in Europe has been primarily on this species. So now, the overwhelming body of medical knowledge on Echinacea is on extracts of E. purpurea, when in fact E. angustifollia was the species that was primarily used in the U.S. during the 1800s and early 1900s.

The demise of Echinacea
Echinacea appeared in the National Formulary until 1947, and the United States Dispensatory until 1943. However, Echinacea, like all botanical medicines, eventually left mainstream medicine. In 1910, botanicals no longer dominated the United States Pharmacopoeia (USP), comprising only 47% of the 773 drugs listed. The Flexner Report, a study of U.S. medical education, unfavorably contrasted botanical based medical establishments with conventional medical school models. Paul Ehrlich's new drug for syphillus, arsphenamine achieved positive results. And, Echinacea, whose therapeutic actions are via a nonspecific stimulation of the immune system, was much less sexy than the direct antimicrobial effects of the new synthetics. Not to mention the fact that the American Medical Association really didn't

want anything to do with Echinacea because it was so strongly identified with the Eclectics.

Science:

Which species is best

Echinacea is a very complicated compound. First of all, most of what we knew about it from a chemical aspect has to be discounted because of the misidentification of Echinacea species prior to 1986. Then, there are eight or more unrelated active chemicals that affect the immune system, in about twenty different ways, but not each of the three species used medicinally have the same chemical makeup. Much of what we know today about Echinacea's chemistry is due to the great work done by Professor H. Wagner at the Institute of Pharmaceutical Biology in Munich, and Professor Rudi Bauer at the Institute of Pharmaceutical Biology at Heinrich-Heine University in Düsseldorf.

For example, the roots and tops of E. purpurea and E. angustifollia, as well as the tops of E. pallida, contain alkylamides, named isobutylamides (for those of you who have ever tasted an Echinacea extract, this is the compound that tingles your tongue). However, the roots of E. pallida have only trace amounts if alkylamides, but instead contain polyacetylenes which are absent in the other two species. Additionally, E. purpurea contains the polypropenoid, cichoric acid, while E. angustifollia and E. pallida's polypropenoid content is dominated by echinacoside, not even present in E. purpurea. And, another polypropenoid, cynarin, can only be found in E. angustifollia. What a mess.

So, what can we take home from this? There are two facts to consider. All three species have immunostimulatory activity. And, no single photochemical can be associated with Echinacea's actions, and activity probably depends on the combined action of several compounds. This might imply that the broader the chemical composition, the greater the effect, based on the possible synergistic effects among constituents. Therefore, the best medicinal preparation might be one that combines all three species. Just a thought.

How does it work?

The primary actions of Echinacea are anti-inflammatory, immunostimulant, antibacterial, and vulnerary (wound healing). Sound and plentiful research has focused on Echinacea's ability to stimulate the immune system. The primary pharmacological effects are:

1. Stimulation of phagocytosis

   Phagocytosis is the process by which foreign cells or particles are ingested.

   Echinacea increases the release and activation of macrophages and subsequently, T lymphocytes, tumor necrosis factor, prostaglandins, and interferons (proteins with antiviral and antitumor activity).

2. Up regulation of cellular respiratory activity.

3. Increased mobility of white blood cells

   Echinacea activates a non-specific immune response via a part of the immune system known as the alternate complement pathway.

4. Inhibition of hyaluronidase

   Hyaluronic acid helps keep tissue intact. Hyaluronidase is an enzyme that attacks hyaluronic acid, making tissue susceptible to attack and ultimately infection.

   Echinacea helps to fight the attacking hyaluronidase, thus protecting healthy tissue from being attacked by invaders. This activity of Echinacea contributes to its wound healing (vulnerary) action, in addition to lessening the spread of infectious agents.

   o Exertion of a mild cortisone-like effect, and enhancement of adrenal cortex hormones. This action appears to be responsible for Echinacea's direct antiinflammatory activity.

Modern Day Uses:

The vast amount of positive outcome clinical studies support the use of Echinacea for:

- ➢ Preventing and treating cold and flu
- ➢ Preventing and treating upper respiratory infections
- ➢ Increasing general immune system function
- ➢ Treating vaginal candidiasis

Echinacea is also often prescribed for:

- ➢ Recurrent ear infections
- ➢ Urinary tract infections
- ➢ Sinus infections
- ➢ Throat infections
- ➢ Antibiotic adjunct therapy
- ➢ Cancer adjunct therapy
- ➢ Rheumatoid arthritis
- ➢ Allergies
- ➢ Psoriasis
- ➢ Burns
- ➢ Herpes
- ➢ Blood or food poisoning
- ➢ Externally for
- • Wound healing
- • Abscesses
- • Boils
- • Burns
- • Eczema
- • Cold sores
- • Herpes
- • Vaginitis
- • Psoriasis
- • Periodontal disease
- • Bites (insect, animal, snake)

Contrary to the autoimmune guidelines (see cautions), one study, reported in 1997, suggests that Echinacea may be useful in the treatment of chronic fatigue syndrome and AIDS. However, until more data becomes available, patients with these disorders should exercise caution.

Dose:

There are so many preparations, using different forms of Echinacea, it's impossible to give any advice on dosage other than to follow the manufacturer's guidelines. I can, however, suggest that Echinacea works best if started at the onset of a cold or the flu. I would take Echinacea for about 10 days, which means that I would continue taking it for several days after symptoms subside.

To ensure that you get a product that is concentrated and can guarantee consistent potency, choose one that has been standardized. Look for actives like echinacosides, cichoric acid, and chlorogneic acid. Generally, a dose of a dry extract would be 300-400mg three times daily on an empty stomach. I usually double up on my dose for the first two days.

There is nothing in the literature to discourage the use of Echinacea during pregnancy and lactation.

Cautions:

No significant side effects have been reported in more than 2.5 million prescriptions per year in Germany and more than a century of use in the United States. If this is not a confirmation of safety, I don't know what is.

I am not an advocate of the prolonged use of Echinacea. I classify this plant as a sickness medicine, not a wellness medicine. I personally use it only at the first sign of illness and continue its use for a reasonable period after the symptoms of the illness have allayed. Exceptions to the rule might include short-term use as a preventative in cases where a family member is ill, or on airline journeys during the cold and flu seasons.

Almost nobody would dream of driving their car cross country, putting the pedal to the metal in California and not letting up until they saw the Atlantic. So, why would you want to do that to your immune system.

Giving your killer system a kick in the rear to jumpstart it is one thing, but driving it into the ground is yet another.

Additionally, because Echinacea is an immune stimulant, it should be avoided by people whose immune system is already out of control, namely those with autoimmune diseases. You know who you are. Keep in mind that this caution is based on a theoretical potential for stimulating the autoimmune process and not hard clinical data. I am not aware of any clinical studies confirming this speculation. Echinacea primarily stimulates phagocytosis. Would phagocytosis aggravate the immune response, or help it? However, those suffering from tuberculosis, leukoses, multiple sclerosis, collagen disorders (like lupus), and other autoimmune diseases should take note.

References:
See General Resources

Awang, D, et al. "Echinacea." *Canadian Pharmaceutical Journal.* 1991; 512-516

Barrett, B. et al. "Echinacea for Upper Respiratory Infection." *J Family Practice.* 48: 628-35 YEAR missing

Bauer, R. "Echinacea: Biological Effects and Active Principles." *Phytomedcines of Europe Chemistry and Biological Activity.* American Chemical Society, Washington DC. 1998

Bone, K. "Echinacea: When Should it be Used?" *The European Journal of Herbal Medicine.* 1998; Winter:13-17

Braunig, B. et al. "Echinacea purpurea Root for Strengthening the Immune Response in Flu-Like Infections." *Zeitschr Phytother.* 1992; 13:7-13

Coeugniet, E. et al. "Recurrent Candidiasis: Adjuvant Immunotherapy with Different Formulations of Echinacin®." *Therapiewoche.* 1986; 36:3352-8

Flannery, M. "From Rudbecia to Echinacea: The emergence of the Purple Cone-flower in Modern Therapeutics." *Pharmacy in History.* 1999; 41:52-59

Hobbs, C. *The Echinacea Handbook.* Eclectic Medical Publications. Portland, OR. 1989

Hobbs, C. *Echinacea: The Immune Her* . Capitola, CA. Botanica Press. 1990

Hoheisel, M, et al. "Echinagard Treatment Shortens the Course of the Common Cold: a Double-blind, Placebo-controlled Clinical Trial. *European Journal of Clinical Research*. 1997; 9:261-268

Melchart, D. et al. "Immunomodulation With Echinacea-A Systematic Review of Controlled Clinical Trials." *Phytomed*. 1994; 1:245-54

O'Hara, M, et al. "A Review of 12 Commonly Used Medicinal Herbs." *Arch Fam Med*. 1998; 7:523-536

Roesler, J. et al. "Application of Purified Polysaccharides from Cell Cultures of the Plant Echinacea purpurea to Test Subjects Mediates Activation of the Phagocytic System." *Int J Immunopharm*. 1991; 13:931-41

Schoneberger, D. et al. "The Influence of Immune Stimulating Effects of Pressed Juice From Echinacea Purpurea on the Course and Severity of Colds." *Forum Immunologie*. 1992; 8:2-12

See, M, et al. "In-vitro Effects of Echinacea and Ginseng on Natural Killer and Antibody Dependent Cell Cytotoxicity in Healthy Subjects and Chronic Fatigue Syndrome and AIDS Patients." *Immunopharmacology*. 1997; 35:229-235

Snow, J. "Echinacea Monograph." *Protocol Journal of Botanical Medicine*. 1997; 2:18-24

Stotzem, C. et al. "Echinacea purpurea on the Phagocytosis of Human Granulocytes." *Med Sci Res*. 1992; 20:717-20

Wagner, H. "Herbal Immunostimulants for the Prophylaxis and Therapy of Colds and Influenza." *Eur J Herbal Med*. 1997; 3:1

Fenugreek

(Trigonella foenum-gracum)

Other Common Names:
Hu Lu Ba, Bird's Foot, Greek Hay-seed, Bockshornsame

Background:
Fenugreek is native to North Africa and countries bordering the eastern Mediterranean. The plant part used as a medicine has generally been the seeds. The Ebers Papyrus of 1500 BC Egypt, lists a preparation of Fenugreek for the skin. *"When the body is rubbed with it, the skin is left beautiful without any blemishes."* The Greek physician, Hippocrates, in the 5th century BC, considered it a valuable soothing herb. Another Greek, Dioscorides, in the 1st century AD, recommended Fenugreek for all types of gynecological problems. Ancient Greeks also used it to scent inferior hay. Nearly all cattle like the flavor of Fenugreek in their forage. That is how it actually got its species name; foenum-gracum means "Greek hay."

Over the millennia, Fenugreek has been used as an aphrodisiac, as a treatment for male impotence, and by the Chinese as a warming agent for the kidneys and reproductive organs. Traditional Chinese Medicine has also enlisted Fenugreek for menstrual pain and menopausal problems related to kidney *qi* (energy) weakness.

In ancient Egypt, Fenugreek was used to ease childbirth and to increase milk flow. Today in Cairo, it is used as a concoction called *Helba* to allay gastric distress, fever, and for diabetes. And, Fenugreek is still used by Egyptian women for menstrual pain.

In this country, for the first half of the 20th century, a preparation called Lydia Pinkham's Vegetable Compound was one of the leaders in the market for female problems. According to the original formula, in her own handwriting, Fenugreek was its principal ingredient.

Over the years, with many of its actions bleeding into modern times, Fenugreek has been used in folk medicine for: boils, diabetes, cellulite, tuberculosis, as an external emollient, as a colon lubricant, for gastric and duodenal ulcers, diverticulosis, dysentery, colitis, diarrhea, constipation, irritable bowel, Crohn's disease, poor appetite, chronic cough, bronchitis, anorexia, to reduce fever, and in Arabian medicine, for "alluring roundness of the female breast."

Science:

Two primary constituents in Fenugreek are key to its medicinal activity. The first is its mucilaginous fiber (up to 50%), which is responsible for its soothing properties, gastrointestinal benefits, and to a certain extent, glucose modulating properties. The second is its saponins (up to 5%), which are responsible for its hormonal and glucose controlling actions.

Other components of Fenugreek include alkaloids, protein, flavonoids, coumarins, lipids, vitamins, and minerals.

Modern Day Uses:

Fenugreek seeds have a taste somewhat reminiscent of maple sugar, and it is still used as a spice and flavoring agent, especially in imitation maple syrup. In the pharmaceutical industry, Fenugreek is currently used as the source of diosgenin, one of its active constituents from which other steroids can be synthesized.

German Commission E approves Fenugreek seeds for the treatment of anorexia, internally, and for local inflammation, topically. In the rest of Europe, Asia, the Middle East, and Upper Africa, Fenugreek is used for many of the traditional indications mentioned above, and for good reasons. For example, a recent study demonstrated that the steroid saponins of Fenugreek enhance food consumption and motivation to eat.

Diabetes and Atherosclerosis

However, some of the traditional uses have prompted numerous clinical studies that may establish historical uses as modern uses, namely hyperlipidemia and diabetes. And then there is the breast thing.

Studies show that Fenugreek significantly lowers blood glucose and plasma glucagon levels. Test results suggest it can improve peripheral glucose utilization, which contributes to improvement in glucose tolerance. Fenugreek appears to exert its hypoglycemic effect by acting at the insulin receptor as well as the gastrointestinal level.

Fenugreek has been shown to exert a cholesterol-lowering effect. In one 24-week study, serum cholesterol, triglycerides, LDL and VLDL levels showed a steady decrease over the testing period. Additionally, HDL levels (good cholesterol) showed a 10% increase. Results like this would indicate Fenugreek could be beneficial in preventing and treating atherosclerosis.

Boobs Boobs Boobs
Fenugreek was once fed to harem women to make them more busty. And, believe it or not, this indication has found its way back onto the American market. According to the highly respected herbalist, James Duke, Ph.D., the seeds and sprouts have a centuries-old folk reputation as breast enlargers. In his book, *The Green Pharmacy*, he states that there are modern testimonials for Fenugreek's effects on breasts, and that he has good reason to believe the herb really works.

Fenugreek does contain diosgenin, a steroid that can be converted into estrogen. Estrogen has many effects on the female body including growth of breast cells, and breast water retention. I do remember, in my pharmacy practice days, many women taking birth-control pills complained about their breasts becoming enlarged and heavy. So maybe, who knows?

Duke also mentions that massaging powdered Fenugreek into the breasts is also worth a try, as breast tissue can apparently absorb a certain amount of plant chemicals. Now, this makes much more sense to me. Even if the treatment doesn't work, one would have had a lot more fun working with one's significant other, trying.

Fenugreek has been used since Biblical times to increase the production of milk for nursing. This action is probably also due to the estrogen-like activity for which the herb is known. It has been my observation that women who use Fenugreek for this purpose report back beneficial and satisfactory results.

Dose:
If you are into taking the seeds, use 1-6 grams three times daily. Otherwise, use Fenugreek seed capsules. Try one to three 500mg capsules three times daily.

Cautions:
Because of possible oxytocic (uterine stimulating) effects Fenugreek may exert, this herb should be avoided during pregnancy, unless otherwise directed by one's physician.

Fenugreek has been shown to have a hypoglycemic effect. That means that if you are taking medicine to lower your blood sugar, the herb could make your drug stronger. Therefore, let your doctor know what you are doing so that he can act accordingly. If you are using insulin, watch your sugar levels more closely.

Fenugreek is very high in fiber. It is not a good idea to take any medication with a fiber supplement due to possible absorption interference. Leave yourself a two-hour window between the time you take your medication and the time you consume Fenugreek.

References:
See General Resources

Duke, J. *The Green Pharmacy*. Emmaus, PA, Rodale Press. 1997

Sharma, R, Sarkar, D., et al. "Hypolipidemic Effect of Fenugreek Seeds: a Chronic Study in Non-Insulin Dependent Diabetic Patients." *Phytotherapy Research* 10:332-334. 1996

Sharma, R, et al. *Phytotherapy Research*. 5:145-147. 1991.

Petit P, at al. "Saponins From Fenugreek Seeds: Extraction, Purification, and Pharmacological Investigation on Feeding Behavior and Plasma Cholesterol. *Steroids* 60:674. 1995

Raghuram, T. et al. Effect of Fenugreek Seeds on Intravenous Glucose Disposition in Non-Insulin Dependent Diabetic Patients. *Phytotherapy Research*. 8:83-6. 1994

Feverfew

(Taracetum parthenium; Chrysanthemum parthenium)

Other Common Names:
Featherfew, Bachelor's Button, Featherfoil, Altamisa, Midsummer
Daisy, Febrifuge Plant, Nosebleed, Santa Maria, Wild Quinine

Background:
Feverfew is a bushy perennial that resembles chamomile and grows
along fields and roads of Europe. It is native to the Balkans, but today,
in addition to Europe, is naturalized in North and South America.
Feverfew is a plant with two valid botanical names. Both Taracetum
and Chrysanthemum are used in influential taxonomic reference
works. This is actually unfortunate because it leads to confusion.

Some sources claim that the name Feverfew comes from the Latin
febrifugia, which means "driver of fevers." However, the plant was
never called *Febrifugia*. The ancient Greeks called it *parthenion*, from
parthenos for virgin, and used it for menstrual problems, not fever.
During the Middle Ages the plant picked up the name Featherfoil,
because of its feather-like leaf borders. Feverfew evolved out of the
name Featherfoil, and use of the herb for fevers started after the name
change.

Because Feverfew is strong smelling, herbalists often planted them
around their homes to purify the air. It was believed that malaria,
which had plagued Europe since prehistoric times, was caused by bad
air. The name malaria comes from the Italian *mala*, meaning foul, and
aria, meaning air. Perhaps Feverfew was tried to lower the fever
associated with malaria based on this association. However, it was not
until Spanish explorers brought cinchona bark back from Peru that a
worthy treatment for malaria was brought on board.

Other traditional uses of Feverfew have included: anemia, earaches,
trauma, parasites, insect repellent, to treat bites and stings, ringing in
ears, vertigo, difficulty during labor, stomach aches, toothaches,
hysterical complaints, nervousness and lowness of spirits, and as a

general tonic. But the doctor with the greatest insight may have been a 17th century Englishman, John Parkinson. He claimed Feverfew to be "effectual for all pains of the head." And Sir John Hill, another famous 18th century physician wrote, "In the worst headache, the herb exceeds whatever else is known."

Use of Feverfew declined over several hundred years until the 1970s when sufferers of migraine headaches and arthritis began using it as an alternative medicine. Feverfew's explosion in popularity can be credited to the wife of the chief medical officer of Britain's National Coal Board. She suffered from chronic migraines until a miner shared his secret of chewing Feverfew leaves. She tried it, got immediate results, and after 14 months, was free of headaches. Her husband was impressed and brought his wife's phenomenon to a Dr. E. Stewart Johnson of the City of London Migraine Clinic, who, in turn, tried it on some of his patients (This wouldn't happen in the U.S.). He was impressed enough with the results that he tried it on another 270 of his patients and surveyed the results. And fine results they were. Seventy percent of the subjects reported significant relief.

What followed was Dr. Johnson arranging for rigorous scientific trials. Tests were double-blind and placebo controlled. Results published in the *British Medical Journal* and *Lancet*, validated Feverfew's value in the treatment of migraines.

Science:

Of late, Feverfew has been extensively studied for the prevention of migraine headaches. We believe that it prevents migraines through its effects on serotonin, a neurotransmitter believed to play an integral role in the headache syndrome. It inhibits the release of serotonin from platelets and other inflammatory cells. Other effects that may contribute to the effectiveness of this plant extract include an inhibition of the synthesis of inflammatory prostaglandins and a reduction of platelet aggregation.

The major active phytochemicals in the plant are sesquiterpene lactones, principally Parthenolide. Recent clinical trials have unearthed two monkey wrenches in the system. First of all, a survey of commercially available Feverfew products discovered that many products contained no Parthenolide at all, and that many contained only trace amounts. This would sound a lot worse if it were not for the fact that current research is discovering that even products with high Parthenolide products aren't always working.

Not all migraines are caused by the same triggers. For those individuals in whom serotonin release is the primary trigger/underlying or initiating mechanism, feverfew could be helpful, but there are at least ten other triggering metabolic dysfunctions for migraine, and it is conceivable that feverfew may not be effective against those.

Or, the conclusion may lie in the chemotype of plant used. The positive British studies were all done with similar plants. No Feverfew extract has thus far been shown to be effective for migraine prevention. A recent Dutch trial done with an extract standardized to the arbitrary .2% Parthenolide standard established, did not yield a positive outcome.

This leaves the consumer out in left field. Until more studies are done to elucidate Feverfew's actives, and identifying the plant varieties that are effective, it is kind of a hit and miss situation. You may have to try different brands before settling on an effective one.

Modern Day Uses:

Feverfew is indicated for the long-term treatment and prevention of migraine headaches. Health Canada, Canada's equivalent to our FDA, has approved feverfew capsules as an over-the-counter medication for migraine prevention. In my opinion, Health Canada lives in the Dark Ages. If they approve Feverfew, it must be very special.

Other contemporary uses of Feverfew might include:

> ➤ Digestive aid- Feverfew is a close relative of Chamomile, and likewise contains phytochemicals that are antispasmodic and soothing to the gastrointestinal tract.

> ➤ Menstrual cramps- Feverfew is a smooth muscle relaxant and blocks prostaglandins linked to pain and inflammation.

> Arthritis- Feverfew suppresses inflammatory prostaglandins, leukotrienes and thromboxanes, three culprits of inflammation. It acts much like nonsteroidal anti-inflammatory drugs, but without the side effects.

> Rheumatoid arthritis- coupled with other actions of Feverfew, is its ability to inhibit the release of inflammatory chemicals from platelets.

Dose:

Until more is learned to uncover Feverfew's mysteries, chose a product prepared from dried leaf, standardized to at least .2% Parthenolide. While Parthenolide may not be the active, at least it is a marker. If you can find Feverfew grown in the U.K., you may improve your chances of effectiveness. In Canada, where Feverfew is an over-the-counter drug for migraines, the recommended dose is 125 mg daily of .2% Parthenolide standardized preparation. This yields a daily intake of 250 micrograms of Parthenolide.

Remember that Feverfew suppresses migraines and is not a cure. It is to be used on a maintenance basis. Feverfew has been shown to decrease the severity, frequency, and duration of headaches. Clinical experience dictates that it may take four to six weeks to effect a positive outcome.

Consider supplementing with vitamin B-2 and magnesium to possibly further enhance the effectiveness of Feverfew. Every little bit helps.

Cautions:

Studies using standardized extract capsules of Feverfew have demonstrated no significant side effects, just a few isolated cases of mild gastrointestinal upset. If you decide to go the route of chewing leaves, consider that 5%-15% of users develop oral ulcers and/or gastrointestinal tract irritation.

During the clinical trials that validated Feverfew's use for migraines, it was noted that the herb also showed a reduction in blood pressure. Based on this, it would make sense that those on standard medical treatment for hypertension monitor their blood pressure closely while using Feverfew. Since Feverfew is a long-term treatment for migraine, one's physician may want to reduce the dose of drug if Feverfew is helping the problem.

Feverfew may increase the risk of bleeding in patients on anticoagulant therapy. Discuss its use with your health care professional before starting the herb.

Sudden discontinuation can precipitate rebound headaches.

References:

See General Resources

Awang, D. "Herbal Medicine, Feverfew." *Can Pharm J.* 1989; 122:26-70

Awang, D. "Prescribing Therapeutic Feverfew." *Integrative Medicine.* 1998; 1:11-13

Barsby, R, et al. "Feverfew and Vascular Smooth Muscle: Extracts from Fresh and Dried Plant Show Opposing Pharmacological Profiles, Dependent Upon Sequiterpene Lactone Content." *Planta Medica.* 1993; 59:20-5

Castleman, M. *The Healing Herbs.* Emmanaus, PA. Rodale Press. 1991

DerMarderosian, A ed. *Review of Natural Products.* St. Louis, MO, Facts and Comparisons, 1999

DeWeerdt, C, et al. "Randomized Double-Blind Placebo Controlled Trial of a Feverfew Preparation." *Phytomedicine.* 1996; 3:225

Ernst, E. the Clinical Efficacy of Herbal Treatments: An Overview of Recent Systematic Reviews. *The Pharmaceutical Journal,* 1999; 262: 85-87

Foster, S. *Feverfew.* American Botanical Council. Botanical Series 310. 1996

Foster, S. "Feverfew: When the Head Hurts." *Alternative & Complimentary* Therapies. 1995; 9/10:35-337

Hepinstall, S, et al. "Parthenolide Content and Bioactivity of Feverfew. Estimation of

Commercial and Authenticated Feverfew Products." *J Pharm Pharmacol*. 1992; 44:391-5

Hepinstall, S, et al. "Extracts of Feverfew Inhibit Granule Secretion in Blood Platelets and Polymorphonuclear Leukocytes." *Lancet*. 1985; 5:1071-4

Johnson, E, et al. "Efficacy of Feverfew as Prophylactic Treatment of Migraine." *British Med J*. 1985; 291:569-73

Murphy, J. et al. "Randomized Double-blind Placebo-controlled Trial of Feverfew in Migraine Prevention." *Lancet*. 1988; 189-92

O'Hara, M, et al. "A Review of 12 Commonly Used Medicinal Herbs." *Arch Fam Med*. 1998; 7:523-536

Palevitch, D, et al. "Feverfew as a Prophylactic Treatment for Migraine: A Double-Blind Placebo Controlled Study." *Phytother Res*. 1997; 11:508-11

Peikert, A, et al. "Prophylaxis of Migraine with Oral Magnesium : Results from a Prospective, Multicenter, Placebo-Controlled Study." *Cephalagia*. 1996; 16:257-63

Garlic

(Allium sativum)

Other Common Names:
Allium, Stinking Rose, Rustic Treacle, Poor Man's Treacle, Nectar of the Gods, Camphor of the Poor, Clove Garlic, Garlic Clove

Background:
Garlic has served man in the function of both food and medicine for, some believe, 6000 years. A member of the lily family, Garlic is cultivated throughout the world.

The use of Garlic is well documented by the Egyptians, Greeks and Romans. It was mentioned in one of the oldest pharmacological documents known, the *Ebers Papyrus* dating to 1500 BC, where Garlic is included in 22 of its 800 therapeutic formulae. The ailments mentioned in the papyrus were heart problems, headache, bites, worms and tumors—some of the same ailments for which Garlic has now been scientifically proven effective. It is said that the builders of the pyramids were paid in the coin of the realm, onions and Garlic, valuable commodities. The Roman herbalist, Pliny the Elder, recommended it to treat asthma, coughs, and parasites, but also warned about two of my favorite side effects: the gastric burn from ordering "excessive" garlic on my food rather than just asking for extra, followed by the special Garlic flatulence.

In India, Garlic was mentioned in the Ayurvedic *Bower Manuscript*, dated about 450 BC. Its indication was as an antiseptic lotion for washing wounds and ulcers. In ancient China, Garlic was traditionally used for fevers, dysentery, and intestinal parasites.

Homer mentions Garlic in his famous *Odyssey*. The athletes of the original Olympic games in ancient Greece traditionally chewed a clove of Garlic before participation in the games. I suspect this tradition was started by the wrestlers. In some parts of Europe, there is still a superstition that if a racer chews a clove of Garlic before the race, it will prevent his competitors from getting ahead of him. Some Hungarian jockeys have been know to attach a clove to the bits of their horses in the belief that the odor will cause others to fall back.

Galen, an early Greek healer, spoke of Garlic as the panacea of the common man. Hippocrates prescribed Garlic for uterine tumors. And, the Vikings and Phoenicians always carried Garlic on their ocean voyages. The Crusaders brought Garlic back to France. The emperor Charlemagne instructed his subjects to cultivate Garlic. King Henry IV was baptized with a clove of Garlic on his lips, and even though he was known to chew a clove of raw Garlic every morning upon arising, never had trouble getting a date. The prophet Mohammed recommended that Garlic be applied to the sting of a scorpion and the bite of a viper.

Garlic is the principle ingredient in the famous *Four Thieves Vinegar*, still available in France today. The way the story goes is that, during the plague in 1722 France, four condemned criminals were recruited to bury the dead. When they proved to be immune to the disease, they confessed that they owed their health to a concoction they consumed that consisted of copious quantities of Garlic in vinegar (or wine).

It has only been in the last 200 years that Garlic has undergone extensive medical study. Known to so many of us as Russian Penicillin, its antimicrobial activity was first clinically reported by Louis Pasteur in 1858. Garlic was used by Albert Schweitzer in Africa to treat dysentery. In 1892, two Germans, Semmler and Welthiem, were able to begin isolating Garlic's actives, namely its sulfur compounds. Since organic sulfur is known to be a universal antiseptic, it comes as no surprise that Garlic was enlisted in WWI as a battle treatment for the prevention of gangrene. The raw juice was expressed, diluted with water, and put on swabs that were applied to the wounds. Its popularity waned with the introduction of new miracle antibiotics. Who knows how many limbs or lives have been saved by the Stinking Rose?

Science:

Garlic contains some unusual sulfur-containing phytochemicals including allicin, allin, scordinin, ajoenes, dithins and diallylsulfides to name only a few. The compound allin has no smell or taste in its steady state. However, as soon as garlic is crushed, sliced, or cut, the allin makes contact with an enzyme, called alliinase, that creates a powerful and highly pungent substance called allicin. Garlic's properties primarily result from allicin and its other phytochemical sulfur compounds. Although allicin is probably the best known, a significant amount of research data exists which reveals the beneficial properties of the other compounds. The primary benefits of dithins and diallylsulfides, however, seem to be as synergists to the other compounds.

Cardiovascular Benefits

Epidemiological studies have noticed an inverse relationship between Garlic consumption and cardiovascular disease. For example, take the data that has emerged from studying the vegetarian Jains of India, some of whom are prohibited from eating Garlic. The study divided subjects into three groups, big, medium and non-Garlic eaters. The group that consumed the most Garlic had the lowest cholesterol levels (159). The group that did not consume Garlic had the highest (209). Your first reaction might be that a total cholesterol of 209 is not bad. It is not, but remember that these are vegetarians. Additionally, the fibrinolytic activity in the blood was inversely proportional to the amount of Garlic consumed. Fibrin is a component in blood involved in clotting.

Studies on high fat, high cholesterol, or high alcohol diets have clearly demonstrated that Garlic can prevent raised serum cholesterol or triglyceride levels. It appears to act both by increasing the excretion of sterols and by suppression of cholesterol and lipid synthesis in the liver. Constituents in Garlic have been shown to block enzymes necessary for lipogensis and cholesterol production. Like many popular drugs used today, they block HMG-CoA (an enzyme necessary for the rate-limiting step of cholesterol production in the liver), and fatty acid synthetase.

Garlic lowers LDL (bad) cholesterol, raises HDL (good) cholesterol, and lowers triglycerides. In individuals with the most severe hyperlipidemia given Garlic, reduction in lipid levels was the most significant. It has also been shown to inhibit LDL oxidation, like vitamin E, thus slowing down the process of atherosclerosis. In a four year study released in 1999, researchers also concluded that Garlic effectively prevented the progression of existing atherosclerotic plaques, and in many cases, actually led to a slight regression in plaque size.

Garlic has also been shown to inhibit platelet aggregation, enhance fibrinolysis, reduce plasma viscosity, increase the activity of nitric oxide sythase (a molecule involved in vasodilitation), and to have a mild blood pressure lowering effect. A study, published in 1997, looked at pulse wave velocity (PWV) and elastic vascular resistance (EVR), measures of arteriosclerosis (hardening of the arteries). After two years of Garlic supplementation, both PWV and EVR were significantly lower in the Garlic group, showing it to have a preventative effect on age-related arterial stiffness.

Cancer
Epidemiological studies have found that populations who eat significant quantities of Garlic have a decreased incidence of many cancers. For example, in one study of 41,837 women, a 35% lower incidence of colon cancer was enjoyed by the subjects who consumed one or more servings of Garlic weekly, and a 50% lower risk of colon cancer was also seen at about this dose.

German scientists reported in 1990 that two of Garlic's components exhibited cytotoxic effects against three cancer cell lines. This was a test tube study but showed that one component, ajoene, was twice as toxic to cancer cells as to normal cells. It would be nice if drugs we use in chemotherapy acted this way.

Antimicrobial
The antimicrobial effect of Garlic is believed to be largely due to its allicin content. Allicin inhibits the growth of both gram-positive and gram-negative bacteria. When used with modern antibiotics, Garlic seems to enhance their effectiveness. Other studies show Garlic to also have anticandidal activity. The use of Garlic with antibiotics is a therapeutic match made in heaven.

Modern Day Uses:
Garlic combines the wisdom of time with modern science. It affords a high level of safety while providing protection against:

> Cardiovascular diseases
> High cholesterol and triglycerides
> Cancer
> Free radicals
> Oxidation
> Radiation
> Pollution
> Immune deficiency
> Viruses
> Intestinal parasites
> Inflammation
> Infection
> Stress
> Fatigue
> Candida
> Ulcers

It seems like everyday we are hearing about new discoveries of the therapeutic benefits of Garlic that may help us to better treat some of today's most devastating and chronic diseases.

Dose:

Many commercially preparations of Garlic are available. Some of these have been "deodorized." Since the antibacterial and anti-lipidemic actions appear to be associated with the odor constituents, the therapeutic value of deodorized Garlic has been questioned. I personally use a product standardized to contain over 7000 mcg allicin (odorous chemical in Garlic).

Another caveat is that the enzyme that converts alliin into the active allicin is inactivated by cooking or acid. If you prefer to eat your medicine, eat it raw. If you prefer to take your medicine in tablet form, look for one that protects the actives from the high acid level of the stomach (pH 1-2) and releases its payload in the non-hostile areas of the GI system (pH 4.5-8).

For those using Garlic therapeutically, consider that some of the better medical studies used 900 mg per day of a product standardized to .6%

allicin. Unfortunately, that meant having to take 9 tablets three times daily. More concentrated products are available. The one I take is also standardized to .6% allicin, but each tablet provides 600 mg of Garlic extract.

Cautions:

Garlic is virtually non-toxic, if you don't consider the effect on your breath, and that is only toxic to your friends. Some people suffer superficial short-lived digestive effects that include, burning, nausea, and gas. With doses equivalent to eating two whole heads of crushed garlic, cases of loss of appetite, vomiting, and diarrhea, and rightfully so, have been reported.

Remember that Garlic is an anticoagulant and could have a synergistic effect on other natural anticoagulants or medications. Don't take anticoagulants before surgery. Garlic has also been shown to reduce blood sugar levels by increasing serum insulin and improving liver glycogen storage. If you are using therapeutic doses of medicinal grade Garlic and suffer from Diabetes, watch your blood sugar tests more closely.

References:

See General Resources

Ali, M. & Thomson, M. "Consumption of a Garlic Clove a Day Could Be Beneficial in Preventing Thrombosis." *Prostagl Leukotrines Essential Fatty Acids*. 1995; 53:211-12

Boullin, D. "Garlic as Platelet Inhibitor." *Lancet*. 1979; I:776-777

Block, E. "The Chemistry of Garlic and Onions." *Scientific American*. 1985; 252:94-99

Cavallito, C, et al. "Allicin, the Antibacterial Principle of Allium Sativum. Isolation, Physical Properties, and Antibacterial Action." *J Am Chem Soc*. 1944; 66:1950-1951

Chang, M, et al. "Effect of Garlic on Carbohydrate Metabolism and Lipid Synthesis in Rats." *J Nutrition*. 1980; 110:931

Cheng, J, et al. "Optimal Dose of Garlic to Inhibit Dimethylhydrazine-Induced Colon Cancer." *World J Surg*. 1995; 19:621-6

Das, I, et al. "Potent Activation of Nitric Oxide Synthase by Garlic: A Basis for its Therapeutic Applications." *Curr Med Research Opinion.* 1995; 13:257-63

Didry, N, et al. "Antimicrobial Activity of Naphthoquinones and Allium Extracts Combined with Antibiotics." *Pharm Acta Helv.* 1992; 67:148-151

Dorant, E. et al. "Garlic and its Significance for the Prevention of Cancer in Humans: A Critical View." *Br J Cancer.* 1993; 67:424-29

Holzgartner, H. et al. "Comparison of the Efficacy and Tolerance of a Garlic Preparation vs. Benzafibrate." *Arzneim Forsch Drug Res.* 1992; 42:1473-7

Hughes, B, et al. "Antimicrobial Effects of Allium Sativum..." *Phytotherapy Research.* 1991; 5:154-158

Jain, A. et al. "Can Garlic Reduce Levels of Serum Lipids? A Controlled Clinical Study." *Am J Med.* 1993; 94:632-5

Kieswetter, H, et al. "Effect of Garlic on Thrombocyte Aggregation, Microcirculation, and Other Risk Factors." *Int J Clin Pharmacol Ther Toxicol.* 1991; 29:151-5

Koscielny, J, et al. "The Antiathersclerotic Effect of Allium Sativum." *Athersclerosis.* 1999; 144:237-49

Kritchevsky, D, et al. "Influence of Garlic Oil on Cholesterol Metabolism in Rats." *Nutrition Reports International.* 1980; 22:641-645

Legnani, C. et al. "Effects of a Dried Garlic Preparation on Fibrinolysis and Platelet Aggregation in Healthy Subjects." *Arzneim Forsch Drug Res.* 1993; 43:119-22

Mader, F. "Treatment of Hyperlipidemia with Garlic-Powder Tablets: Evidence fro the German Association of General Practitioners' Multicenter Placebo-Controlled Double-Blind Study." *Arzneim Forsch Drug Res.* 1990; 40:1111-6

Nagourney, R. "Garlic: Medicinal Food or Nutritious Medicine?" *Journal of Medicinal Food.* 1998; 1:13-28

Qureshi, A, et al. "Suppression of Avian Hepatic Lipid Metabolism by Solvent Extract of Garlic: Impact on Serum Lipids." *J Nutrition.* 1983; 113: 1746-1755.

Reuter, H. "Allium Sativum and Allium Ursinum: Part 2 Pharmacology and Medicinal Application. *Phytomedicine.* 1995; 2:73-91

Sainani, G, et al. "Effect of Dietary Garlic and Onion on Serum Lipid Profile in a Jain

Community." *Indian J Med Research.* 1979; 69:776-780

Scharfenberg, K, et al. *Cancer Letters.* 1990; 53:103-8

Sendl, A. "Allium Sativum and Allium Ursinum: Part 1: Chemistry, Analysis, History, Botany."
Phytomedicine; 4:323-39

Silagy, C, et al. "A Meta-Analysis of the Effect of Garlic on Blood Pressure." *J Hypertension.* 1994; 12:463-8

Sok Won Han, et al. *Bulletin of Clinical Research CMC.* 1990; 18:223-236

Vorberg, G, et al. "Therapy with Garlic Results of a Placebo Controlled, Double-Blind Study." *Brit J Clin Prac.* 1990; 44:7

Warshafsky, S. et al. "Effect of Garlic on Total Serum Cholesterol: A Meta-Analysis." *Ann Int Med.* 1993; 119:599-605

Ginger

(Zingiber officinale)

Other Common Names:

Jamaica Ginger, African Ginger, Cochin Ginger, Black Ginger, Race Ginger, Gingembre

Background:

To most of us in the United States, Ginger is a popular seasoning, but for literally thousands of years, it has been used as a medicine in addition to a wonderful food enhancer. The botanical name Zingiber is derived from the ancient Hindu language meaning "horn-shaped" in reference to the protuberances on the root, which is the part of the plant used both in cooking and in medicine. Technically, however, it is the knotted and branched rhizome (underground stem) that is really used, even though we commonly call it the root.

Cultivated for thousands of years in both China and India, the plant is not known in the wild, and its exact origin is not clear. We know that Ginger reached the West a couple of thousand years ago from tax records left behind by the Romans. The Greeks and Romans thought Ginger came from an Arabian region because it was imported from India across the Red Sea. We also know that Ginger was traded into Europe about 800 years ago because of duty records dating back to 1228.

Ginger in China

In China, dried Ginger, known as Gan-jiang is mentioned in the earliest of herbals, *She Nung Ben Cao Jing*, attributed to Emperor Shen Nung, about 2000 BC. Legend has it that Nung, by inventing the cart and plow, taming the ox and yoking the horse, and teaching his people to clear the land with fire, reputedly established a stable agricultural society in China. The *She Nung Ben Cao Jing,* his catalog of 365 species of medicinal plants, became the basis of later herbological studies. Chinese records dating from the 4th century BC indicate that Ginger was used to treat numerous conditions including stomachache, diarrhea, nausea, cholera, hemorrhage, rheumatism, and toothaches.

The Chinese believe that much of Ginger's powers come from its ability to bring fluids to an area, warming it up. They say that it can mobilize the body's defenses. Through its thermogenic action, heat is produced along with more secretions and sweating, which drives out toxins and microbes. Immunity is increased due to the presence of more white cells, and better circulation spreads the improved healing powers throughout the body.

In modern China, in addition to being an essential ingredient in almost every culinary dish, Ginger is used in about half of all herbal prescriptions. One of the main reasons it is added to so many Chinese medicinal mixtures is its ability to act as the "messenger" or "servant" or "guide" herb that brings other herbal medicines to the site where they are needed. In India, studies are showing that adding Ginger to certain drugs can enhance the absorption of the medication. One day, this may lead to Ginger being used for a biopotentiation effect.

Ginger in the United States

The Spaniards transplanted Ginger from the East Indies to Spain and then later, after the discovery of America, naturalized it here. It was popularized by the Eclectic school of medicine around the turn of the 20th century, as exemplified by the following excerpts from an 1898 medical journal. *"This remedy is so common that many of our text books do not deign to mention it; however, it is an excellent remedy and should have a place beside the capsicum bottle on the shelf of every dispensary. It is classified as a stimulant, carminative, dia-phoretic, errhine* (promotes nasal discharge), *sialagogue* (promotes salivation), *rubefacient* (a counterirritant like muscle rubs), *etc."*

"It is pungent, aromatic, and grateful to the taste." "...we believe this remedy is a neglected one. Many times it could be given with, or in alteration with, other remedies to advantage..." "It is a stimulant to the digestive tract, and after all, everything depends upon digestion and assimilation. This tract is to the body what the firebox is to the engine; not enough fire and fuel, not enough steam; not enough food and absorption, not enough blood, or life." "It promotes digestion by stimulation; it removes or prevents flatulence, thereby relieving or overcoming spasm and colic."

"...assists in promoting the secretions and in reducing high temperature, etc. In atonic dyspepsia and enfeebled states of the alimentary tract, with specific nux vomica, ignatia, etc, or with so called bitter tonics if you prefer them, Ginger is an excellent remedy. In diarrhoea, in cholera morbus, with nausea and vomiting, with cold extremities and surface of the body, don't forget Ginger."

It is interesting to note that almost all the benefits of Ginger reported in this journal have been validated by modern science. Crude Ginger, Ginger extracts, and Ginger oleoresin were formerly official drugs of the *United States Pharmacopoeia* and *National Formulary* as a carminative, aromatic and stimulant. In another official compendium of yesteryear, the *King's American Dispensatory*, Ginger was indicated for loss of appetite, flatulence, stomach gurgling, spasmodic gastric and intestinal contractions, and coldness of the extremities. Today, Ginger is official in the pharmacopoeias of many countries. In the Chinese pharmacopoeia, Ginger is listed as an approved drug for epigastric pain with cold feeling, vomiting and diarrhea accompanied by cold extremities and faint pulse, dyspepsia, and cough. The Ayurvedic pharmacopoeia additionally lists it for flatulence and intestinal colic.

Science:

The characteristic odor of Ginger is due to its volatile oils (1-3%), the principal components of which are sesquiterpenes (bisabolene, zingiverene, and zingiberol). However, it is the oleo-resin (mixture of volatile oil and resin) components which are considered the main active principles in Ginger and documented pharmacological actions of these actives generally support the traditional uses. These oleo-resins, sometimes called aromatic ketones, are known collectively as gingerols. They include: 6-gingerol, 6-shogaol, dehydrogingerdione, gingerdione, and zingerone. Commercial Ginger products are standardized to levels of gingerol, the 5% range being considered a good benchmark.

Gingerols have been found to posses cardiotonic as well as antipyretic (fever lowering), analgesic, antitussive (cough inhibiting), and sedative properties when administered to laboratory animals. Shogoals are considered to be twice as pungent as gingerols.

Anti-inflammatory and analgesic actions
Gingerols are also modulators of prostaglandins. They are potent inhibitors of prostaglandin and leukotriene synthesis, through the blocking of prostaglandin synthetase, explaining Ginger's use as an anti-inflammatory agent. They simultaneously reduce specific inflammatory prostaglandins while allowing the maintenance of other prostaglandins that provide systemic protection to remain engaged.

Additionally, studies show that Ginger can improve joint movement in patients with rheumatoid arthritis via a dual inhibition of cyclo-oxygenase (COX) and lipoxygenase pathways. Other studies suggest that Ginger acts as a pain reliever, which is not a giant leap of faith considering that some of its components have structural similarities to other analgesics, for example, aspirin. In fact, Shogaol has been shown to inhibit the release of substance P, like aspirin and cayenne. Ginger can also reduce fever like aspirin can.

Circulatory actions
I believe that the jury is still out on the cardiovascular benefits of Ginger. It is reported to inhibit platelet aggregation. It is supposed to do this by blocking thromboxane formation and proaggregatory prostaglandins. For example, in a study of seven women, 5 grams of raw Ginger reduced thromboxane B-2 concentrations, thus indicating a reduction of platelet aggregation. However, more recent studies with powdered Ginger concluded that it did not reduce thromboxane.

On the other hand, Ginger seems to be beneficial at impairing cholesterol absorption as well as stimulating the conversion of cholesterol to bile acids. By impairing absorption and promoting excretion of blood fats, Ginger could contribute to reducing a major risk associated with cardiovascular disease.

Digestive system actions
Ginger can simultaneously improve gastric motility while exerting antispasmodic effects. That is, it increases motility, but decreases the amplitude of contractions. This is consistent with its use as a gastrointestinal tonic. It stimulates digestion by virtue of its aromatic

bitter activity. It keeps the intestinal muscles toned and eases material through the digestive system. It is also interesting to note that Ginger can prevent ulcer formation due to ethanol, the anti-inflammatory drugs, indomethacin and aspirin, and other common ulcer causing compounds.

Anti-nausea and anti-vomiting actions

I don't think that there is any doubt that Ginger is effective against nausea and vomiting. What is left to determine is the mechanism of action. Does it work only on the gut, blocking GI reactions and subsequently nausea feedback? Or is there an effect on the central nervous system, or both?

The landmark study on Ginger's antiemitic effect was reported in *Lancet*. It compared the effectiveness of Ginger against the drug dimenhydrinate, which puts most people straight to sleep. Ginger outperformed the drug with no side effects and became famous overnight.

Since the time of the *Lancet* report, many more studies have been performed for a variety of conditions which cause nausea and vomiting. One such study was even performed on women with hyperemesis gravidarum, severe vomiting during pregnancy that can result in hospitalization. In that study, over 70% of the women tested preferred Ginger treatment as their choice for relief.

Antibiotic actions

There is still much to be studied on this action, but in a closed system, the volatile oils of Ginger have been shown to inhibit the growth of bacteria. It has been used to kill parasites, and I wonder if this is the reason it is served with sushi. Additionally, in China, it is used as pesticide against aphids and fungal spores.

Other actions of Ginger include thermogenic properties that account for its ability to warm the body and explain its historical use as a diaphoretic. Another historical activity, namely its ability to curb coughs, has been explained by studies that show shogaol to have an effect on par with codeine.

Modern Day Uses:

While Ginger will prove to be valuable for the treatment of multiple problems, the overwhelming scientific support is weighted to pro-digestion and its antiemetic actions. Other applications may include its use in arthritic conditions, cold and flu, and as a supportive herb in botanical combination therapies.

Digestive uses

Consider Ginger as a stimulant of digestion. Consider it if you are having problems with gas; use it as an antispasmodic, if you have problems digesting fats, or having problems with appetite, or just an ordinary stomachache.

Nausea and vomiting

Many clinical trials support the use of Ginger against nausea and vomiting, both prophylactically and acutely, from a variety of causes, including motion sickness, perioperative anesthesia, morning sickness, flu, and even drug side-effects.

About one-third of all people receiving anesthesia for surgery suffer from postoperative nausea and vomiting. Because of all the complications that can occur after surgery, giving less drugs is better than giving more drugs, and there isn't an available anti-nausea medication that is both effective and has no side effects. Unless we dig it out of our garden, that is. Ginger (500 mg orally) was shown to be effective when administered prior to surgery. In fact, none of the subjects tested, in a 1990 study, required postoperative treatment for nausea or vomiting. This was not even the case with the drug against which Ginger was tested.

Some Chinese cooks keep a small piece of Ginger in their mouth to prevent nausea from strong cooking odors. And, not that I would ever endorse overindulgence in alcohol, but if it occurs, add some Ginger to you hangover treatment.

Other uses

Ginger tea is often used for colds and flu. It can produce perspiration and increase circulation, thus potentially helping to speed the removal of toxins from the body. Ginger may also help with the pain and inflammation of diseased joints. It works topically and could be considered a valuable ingredient in a pain rub. And, don't be afraid to try Ginger for any of its other folkloric uses. It can't hurt and may help.

Dose:

Generally speaking, I recommend taking 500mg capsules of powdered Ginger, preferably standardized to around 5% gingerols. Take 1-2 capsules three times daily before meals. If you are using Ginger to prevent motion sickness, start using it a couple of days before your trip.

Cautions:

Considering that Ginger is used globally as a flavoring agent, and is sold as a supplement in every health store, and probably every pharmacy in the U.S. and Europe, there are little, if any, reports of toxicity or adverse effects attributed to it in the medical literature.

Theoretically, components of Ginger could interfere with the drug management of some disease states. Based on Ginger's long safety record, the clinical significance of any interactions is probably negligible, but I always believe that one should err on the side of safety. Based on speculation, if you are taking drugs for your heart or blood pressure, or if you are on anticoagulant therapy, and begin to suffer new or unusual side effects from your medication, discontinue the Ginger. Consult with you health care professional and regroup.

Ginger may improve the absorption of some drugs, making them more effective, but may increase the rate at which the body excretes them, which may play havoc with a dosing regimen. Pay close attention to your body if you take prescription medication and start taking Ginger.

Ginger may increase bile flow, so long-term use may not be appropriate for those who suffer from, or are prone to, gallstones.

References:
See General Resources

Bensky, D, et al. *Chinese Herbal Medicine: Materia Medica*. Seattle, WA. Eastland Press. 1986

Bloyer, W. "Zingiber." *Eclectic Medical Journal*. 1896; 56:342-343

Bone, M, et al. "Ginger Root-A New Antiemetic. The Effect of Ginger Root on Postoperative Nausea and Vomiting After Major Gynecological Surgery. *Anaesthesia*. 1990; 45:669-71

Chang, C, et al. "The Effect of Chinese Medicinal Herb Zingiber Rhizoma Extract on Cytokine Secretion by Human Peripheral Blood Mononuclear Cells." *J Ethnopharmcol*. 1995; 48:13-9

ESCOP, *Monographs on the Medicinal Use of Plant Drugs*. Exeter, England. ESCOP Secretariat. 1997

Ernst, E. "The Clinical Efficacy of Herbal Treatments: An Overview of Recent Systematic Reviews." *The Pharmaceutical Journal*, 1999 262: 85-87

Fischer-Rasmussen, W, et al. "Ginger Treatment of Hyperemsis Gravidarum." *Eur J Obstet Gynecol Reprod Biol*. 1991; 38:19-24

Fulder, S. *Ginger, The Ultimate Home Remedy*. London. Avery Press. 1996

Grontved, A, et al. "Ginger Root Against Seasickness. A Controlled Trial on the Open Sea." *Acta Otolaryngol*. 1988; 105:45-9

Guh, J, et al. "Antiplatelet Effect of Gingerol Isolated from Zingiber Officinale." *J Pharm Pharmacol*. 1995; 47:329-32

Janssen, P, et al. "Consumption of Ginger Does Not Affect *In Vivo* Platelet Thromboxane Production in Humans." *Eur J Clin Nutr*. 1996 50:772-4

Mascolo, N, et al. "Ethnopharmacologic Investigation of Ginger." *J Ethnopharmacol*. 1989; 27:129-40

Micklefield, G, et al. "Effects of Ginger on Gastroduodenal Motility." *Int J Clinical Ther*. 1999; 37:341-6

Mowrey, D, et al. "Motion Sickness Ginger and Psychophysics." *Lancet*. 1982; 1:655-657

O'Hara, M, et al. "A Review of 12 Commonly Used Medicinal Herbs." *Arch Fam*

Med. 1998; 7:523-536

Phillips, S, et al. "Zingiber Officinale An Antiemetic For Day Case Surgery." *Anaesthesia.* 1993; 48:715-7

Srivastava, K, et al. "Ginger and Rheumatic Disorders." *Med Hypotheses.* 1989; 29:25-8

Srivastava, K, et al. "Ginger and Rheumatism and Musculoskeletal Disorders." *Med Hypotheses.* 1992; 39:342-8

Suekawa, M, et al. "Pharmacological Studies on Ginger. I. Pharmacological Actions of Pungent Constituents 6-Gingerol and 6-Shogaol." *J Pharm Dyn.* 1984; 7:836-48

Yamahara, J, et al. "Inhibition of Cytotoxic Drug Induced Vomiting in Suncus By a Ginger Constituent." *J Ethnopharmacol.* 1989; 27:353-5

Ginkgo

(Ginkgo biloba)

Other Common Names:
Maidenhair Tree, GBE, Fossil Tree

Background:
The Ginkgo tree is the world's oldest living tree species. In fact, it is the longest living plant on earth. It has been traced through fossils back 200 million years. That is why it is often referred to as the living fossil.

The Ginkgo species was almost destroyed during the Ice Age, with the exception of some areas in China and Asia. It was then considered a sacred tree and planted around Buddhist Temples. The use of the leaves of the Ginkgo tree can be traced in China for 5000 years. The tree is mentioned in *Sehn Nung Ben Cao Jing*, China's oldest herbal. The leaves were used, as they are today, for their ability to benefit the brain, and for relieving the symptoms of asthma and coughs. In modern China, tablets or injectable drug forms are even used in the treatment of angina pectoris, chronic bronchitis, and high blood fats. A tea made of boiled leaves is still a treatment for frostbite.

The first Westerner to observe Ginkgo was a German surgeon working for the Dutch East India Company in the early 1700s. He called it "Ginkgo" because that is what the Japanese word for it sounded like. In 1771, when botanical names were being given out, the father of plant organization, Linnaeus, assigned it the name Ginkgo Biloba.

Ginkgo was introduced into this country in 1784 for ornamental reasons. Today, it has become a popular urban tree in cities around the world because of its resistance to insects and disease. Some Ginkgo trees even survived the nuclear attack on Hiroshima. I suspect the Ginkgo tree will even make it through our high tech air pollution, long after we do not.

Since 1970, over 400 clinical research studies have been done on extracts derived from Ginkgo leaves, and standardized Ginkgo Biloba Extract (GBX) has become a widely prescribed medicine in Europe. By 1989, over 10 million prescriptions had been written for GBX by over 100,000 doctors around the world. Since, as we age, blood flow can decrease as much as 20%, and Ginkgo is known for increasing blood flow to the brain, "baby boomers" are creating an even greater demand for it.

Science:

What is in Ginkgo?

From a chemistry standpoint, Ginkgo is very interesting. It contains phytonutrients which include flavonoids like kaempferol, quercetin, isorhamnetine, sciadopitysin, luteolin, delphidenon, and procyanidin; organic acids like hydroxykynurenic acid, pyrocatchuic acid, and vanillic acid; and terpene lactones called Ginkgolides and bilobalide. Ginkgolides are not found in any other plant species. It is the Ginkgolides (mainly Ginkgolide B) that are responsible for the circulation activity that Ginkgo possesses. Ginkgolide B inhibits something called PAF (platelet activating factor), which I shall discuss in more detail because it is this activity for which Ginkgo has become so famous. However, the flavonoids should not be considered chopped liver, as it is this family of chemicals that give Ginkgo its antioxidant powers. It is interesting to note that, as with many plants, single isolated components do not provide the activity of the whole extract. This leads one to deduce that it is a pharmacological synergistic blend of chemicals that imparts activity rather than isolated biological actives. This is what makes Nature so fascinating.

What about PAF?

PAF is a phospholipid mediator released from cell membranes by enzymes that causes platelet stickiness, arterial thrombosis, acute inflammation, allergic reactions, and a myriad of other effects on the cardiovascular system by binding with specific receptor sites. Ginkgo's terpene lactones inhibit PAF by competitive antagonism at the PAF membrane receptor site. What that means clinically is natural blood thinning and improved blood flow, prevention of clots in vessels, a reduction of pro-inflammatory functions of the immune system, an inhibition of bronchial constriction and hypersensitivities which can trigger asthma, and an inhibition of cell activation which can trigger blood vessel spasm.

Free radical scavenging

The second most important effect of Ginkgo on vascular membranes is the scavenging of oxygenated free radicals during metabolism. Under normal conditions, this job is handled by the key enzymes superoxide dismutase and glutathione peroxidase. However, during conditions of poor circulation, these natural defenders are overwhelmed and the result is damage to vascular tissues. Antioxidants can absorb reactive toxic substances which would otherwise cause damage to cells and DNA.

Other significant clinical actions

Ginkgo maintains both venous and arterial tone. Venous, via its ability to stimulate release and inhibit the breakdown of catacholamines, which are stimulating neurotransmitters. Arterial, via its ability to simulate prostacyclin and EDRF (endothelium-derived relaxing factor), two potent vasodilators. Ginkgo makes blood vessels more flexible, in addition to the red blood cells that must squeeze through tight capillaries. The combination of these activities makes it easier for blood and hence oxygen, to reach the brain and extremities or anyplace else with fine blood vessels, for example, the eyes or ears.

Ginkgo normalizes cerebral metabolism in ischemic conditions (local anemia due to obstruction, like atherosclerosis, causing arterial narrowing and decreased blood supply). It increases brain glucose consumption and limits electrolyte imbalances.

The last major clinical action of Ginkgo is an increase in the brain of acetylcholine receptor sites and norepinephrine turnover. Acetylcholine is the key neurotransmitter involved in memory, long-term planning, mental focus, concentration, and learning. A deficiency of acetylcholine results in states such as forgetfulness. Acetylcholine is also involved with primitive drives and emotions. In the brain, norepinephrine is involved in learning and memory. A deficiency of norepinephrine can result in depression. It is interesting to note that reduced acetylcholine activity appears to contribute to age-related cognitive

disorders, and that concentrations of norepinephrine in some areas of
the brain are reduced in patients with Alzheimer's disease.

Modern Day Uses:
What can Ginkgo do for you?
Well, if you wanted to paint with the broadest of stokes, you could say
that Ginkgo can be used against the symptoms of aging. Clinical
research reports a clear relationship between Ginkgo and brain function which includes: increased short term memory and increased
mental acuity (a loss of both are symptoms associated with cognitive
decline experienced by the elderly); decreased progression of
Alzheimer's; decreased progression of senility; an elevation in mood
and attitude and lessening in depression; an increase in concentration;
and a lowering in the incidence, severity and duration of headaches,
especially migraines.

In terms of short-term memory gains, we used to think that Ginkgo
worked only on older individuals who were showing signs of reduced
blood flow due to aging. However, new clinical evidence shows that
Ginkgo may even help younger subjects. One study tested healthy
volunteers between the ages of 30 and 59. The conclusion was that
Gingko aided concentration, focus, and alertness. This data is preliminary; larger studies and more sensitive cognitive tests need to be
developed. Take note that the over 50 crowd still benefited more.

Ginkgo is also beneficial to the circulation of the rest of the body.
Medical studies show us that Ginkgo is helpful in the treatment of a
variety circulatory insufficiencies like pain and numbness to the hands
and feet (Raynaud's Syndrome), numbness, tingling, dizziness (vertigo), intermittent claudicaton, ringing in the ears (tinnitis), hearing
loss and deteriorating vision in the elderly (senile cataracts, macular
degeneration, diabetic retinopathy), hemorrhoids, and perhaps even
high blood pressure and heart pain (angina).

Ginkgo Biloba helps keep the blood from over clotting and is useful as
a natural blood thinner. In fact, in Germany, Gingkot is used more
than aspirin for that reason. And, because of its antioxidant activity,
Ginkgo also helps keep brain cells from being damaged by environ-

mental pollution.

A steady stream of clinical studies continue to publicize the benefits of Ginkgo

Ginkgo has been used for lung disorders by the Chinese for thousands of years. However, in a recent study using Ginkgo in the treatment of bronchial asthma, researchers noted a statistically significant improvement in symptoms in only eight weeks of treatment. The symptoms they observed included wheezing, coughing, chest distress, quality of sleep, and the ability to perform various activities. This is another case of modern science validating a traditional use of a plant medicine.

Ginkgo appears to be effective for the sexual dysfunction caused by antidepressants. Selective serotonin reuptake inhibitors (SSRIs) all too often cause sexual problems like decreased libido, erectile difficulties, delayed or lack of orgasm, and ejaculatory failure. A group of men and women received 120 mg of Gingko twice daily for four weeks and experienced alleviation of their problems with an 84% success rate. Additionally, 91% of the women and 76% of the men became a little less depressed.

With the release of Viagra, erectile dysfunction has come out of the closet. Based on clinical trials, Ginkgo might be considered the first line of defense for restoring some life between the sheets. In a recent trial, two groups of men with proven arterial erectile impotence were given 240 mg of Ginkgo for nine months. One group had previously responded to drug injections to the penis, the other group had not. In the first group, all patients regained sufficient erections after six months of treatment. The second group showed improved blood flow and rigidities at six and nine months. Of this group, two-thirds responded to drug therapy after the Ginkgo treatment, and one-third remained impotent (but had a better memory).

Then there is the study that is dear to my heart, and the one I came across in time to add Gingko to my training for a mountaineering trek in the Andes. In a study of mountain climbers on a Himalayan expedition, Ginkgo was found to prevent acute altitude sickness and cold-related vascular problems. The results were that none of the climbers

taking Ginkgo got sick, while 41% of those who took a placebo did.
In my personal trial, I took 100 mg of Ginkgo twice daily and climbed
to 19,000 feet without getting sick. That is not to say that I felt like
dancing a jig up there, and I did, on occasion, suffer from shortness of
breath. What I did not have was headache, dizziness, nausea or vomiting. I also suffered no microcirculation problems like numbness,
tingling, aching of my extremities, or loss of manual dexterity. I also
did not get out of my clothes for 2 ½ weeks, and as a result, some sort
of sexual dysfunction might have been prevented, had the occasion
arisen, but we'll never know.

Dose:

People always ask me which Ginkgo to buy. The answer is simple.
There is only one Ginkgo that I know of that today's medical research
is based on. Any other Ginkgo is virtually absent of scientific support.
And, you can find it in your local vitamin store. Read the label. It
should say each of the following: 50:1 extract, 24% flavonglycosides,
and a minimum of 6% terpene lactones. The 6% terpene lactones is
the most critical measurement, as this is where the Ginkgolide B will
be. Check to see if there is a minimum of .8% Ginkgolide B claimed
on the label. If so, you are probably all right.

The second most frequently asked question I hear is how much should
one take. If you have the real stuff, you should take 120mg to 240mg
daily in divided doses, depending on your own health and needs. I
take 100 mg. twice daily. Higher doses are sometimes used to improve
memory and cognition, but this is O.K. as Ginkgo is very well tolerated even at higher doses. What is just as important as how much, is
how long. Ginkgo should be taken for a minimum of 12 weeks. The
longer the treatment, the more obvious and lasting the results.

Cautions:

Ginkgo is extremely well tolerated. In a retrospective analysis of
reported side effects, only 33 out of 8505 reported untoward effects,
and those were mild and transient problems involving GI upset.

Because of Ginkgo's vascular effects, one might expect it to reduce
blood pressure and perhaps interfere with blood pressure medication.

However, according to the literature, doses of 120mg for six to twelve months had no significant effect on blood pressure. It is not until doses of 360mg daily that effects on blood pressure are noted. Nonetheless, it is better to be cautious and monitor your blood pressure more closely if you are on hypotensive medication and begin to take Ginkgo.

Since Ginkgo is an effective anticoagulant in its own right, it should be used with caution by those taking other anti coagulants or anti platelet agents to avoid bleeding complications. Perhaps one may require a lower dose of medication if using an effective form of Ginkgo. One's health care professional should be part of that decision making process.

As with any agent that affects blood coagulation time, do not take Gingko if you are planning to have surgery.

I am often asked if it is advisable to give a child Ginkgo for memory or concentration problems. My answer is that I am not aware of any studies with children and Ginkgo. Ginkgo benefits the brain mainly through increased blood flow to the brain. A child is more likely to have issues other than circulation causing concentration problems.

References:
See General Resources

Barth, S, et al. "Influences of Ginkgo Biloba on Cyclosporine A Induced Lipid Peroxidation in Human Liver Microsomes in Comparison to Vitamin E, Glutathione and N-Acetylcysteine." *Biochemical Pharmacology.* 1991; 41:1521-26

Boudouresques, G, et al. "Value of Ginkgo Biloba Extract in Cerebrovascular Pathology." *Medecine Practicienne.* 1975; 598:75-78

Braquet, P. "The Ginkgolides: Potent Platelet Activating Factor Antagonists Isolated From Ginkgo Biloba L: Chemistry, Pharmacology, and Clinical Applications." *Drugs of the Future.* 1987; 12:642-88

Braquet, P, et al. "Involvement of Platelet Activating Factor in Respiratory Anaphylaxis, Demonstrated by PAF Acether Inhibitor BN 52021. *Lancet.* 1985; 1:1501

Choussat, H, et al. "Clinical Trial of a Concentrated Vegetable Extract in Geriatrics." *Geriatrie.* 1977; 2:370-75

Cohen, A, et al. "Ginkgo Biloba For Antidepressant-Induced Sexual Dysfunction." *J Sex Marital Therapy*. 1998; 24:139-45

Chung, K, et al. "Effect of Ginkgolide Mixture BN 52063 in Antagonizing Skin and Platelet Responses to Platelet Activating Factor in Man." *Lancet*. 1987; 1:248-51

Cory, E, et al. "Total Synthesis of Ginkgolide B." *B J Am Chem Soc.* 1988; 110:649-651

Drieu, K. "Multiplicity of Effects of Ginkgo Biloba Extract: Current Status and New Trends." *B J Am Chem Soc.* 1985; 63-68

Ernst, E. "The Clinical Efficacy of Herbal Treatments: An Overview of Recent Systematic Reviews." *The Pharmaceutical Journal*, 1999; 262: 85-87

Heiss, W, et al. "The Influence of Drugs on Cerebral Blood Flow." *Pharmakotherapie*. 1978; 1:137-44

Hofferberberth, B. "The Efficacy of Egb761 in Patients with Senile Dementia of the Alzheimer Type, a Double-blind, Placebo-controlled Study on Different Levels of Investigation. *Human Phychopharm*. 1994; 9:215-22

Itil, T, et al. "Central Nervous System Effects of Ginkgo Biloba, a Plant Extract." *Am J Ther*. 1996; 3:63-73

Kanowski, S, et al. "Proof of Efficacy of the Ginkgo Biloba Special Extract Egb 761 in Outpatients Suffering From Mild to Moderate Primary Degenerative Dementia of the Alzheimer Type or Multi-infarct Dementia. *Pharmacopsychiatry*. 1996; 29:47-56

Li, M, et al. "Clinical Observation of the Therapeutic Effect of Ginkgo Leaf Concentrate Oral Liquor on Bronchial Asthma." *CJIM*. 1997; 3:264-7

LeBars, P. et al. "A Placebo-Controlled, Double-Blind, Randomized Trial of an Extract of Ginkgo Biloba for Dementia." *JAMA*. 1997; 278:1327-1332

Mouren, X, et al. "Study of the Anti-Ischemic Action of EGb761 in the Treatment of Peripheral Arterial Occlusive Disease by TcPO2 Determination." *Angiology*. 1994; 45:413-7

Pittler, M, et al. "Ginkgo Biloba Extract for the Treatment of Intermittent Claudication: A Meta-Analysis of Randomized Trials." *Am J Med*. 2000; 108:276-81

Rigney, U, et al. "The Effects of Acute Doses of Standardized Ginkgo Biloba Extract on Memory and Psychomotor Performance in Volunteers." *Phytotherapy Res*. 1999; 13:408-15

Roncin, J, et al. "EGb 761 in Control of Acute Mountain Sickness and Vascular Reactivity to Cold Exposure." *Aviation Space Envrion Med.* 1996; 67:445-452

Schubert, H, et al. "Depressive Episode Primarily Unresponsive to Therapy in Elderly Patients: Efficacy of Ginkgo Biloba Extract in Combination With Antidepressants." *Geriatr Forsch.* 1993; 3:45-53

Sohn, M, et al. "Ginkgo Biloba Extract in the Therapy of Erectile Dysfunction." *J Sex Educ Ther.* 1991; 17:53-61

Stalleicken, D, et al. "Continuous Observation of Cognitive Deficits. Results of a Multicenter Study Conducted on the Basis of Psychological Tests." *Therapiewoche.* 1988; 2:1-8

Taylor, J. "The Effects of Chronic, Oral Ginkgo Biloba Extract Administration on Neurotransmitter Receptor Binding in Young and Aged Fisher 344 Rats." *Effects of Ginkgo Biloba Extract on Cerebral Impairment.* 1985; 31-34

Wettstein, A. "Cholinesterase Inhibitors and Ginkgo Extracts- Are They Comparable in the Treatment of Dementia? Comparison of Published Placebo-Controlled Efficacy Studies of at Least Six Months Duration." *Phytyomed.* 2000; 6:393-401

Witte, S, et al. "Modifications of Viscoelastic Properties During Cardiovascular Diseases." *Clinical Hemorpheology.* 1989; 9:831-37

Ginseng

(Panax quinquefolium; Panax ginseng)

Other Common Names:

P. ginseng: Asian Ginseng, Korean Ginseng, Chinese Ginseng, Panax, Panax Ginseng, Oriental Ginseng, Ginseng Root, Ginseng Radix, Oriental Ginseng, Ren Shen, Seng, Korean Red, Ninjin, Ginseng Asiatique

P. quinquefolium: American Ginseng, Western Ginseng, Rhen Shen, Five Fingers, Tartar Root, Red Berry, Wisconsin Ginseng, Tienchi Ginseng, Sang, Ontario Ginseng, North American Ginseng, Canadian Ginseng, Anchi Ginseng

Background:

What most people refer to as Ginseng is one of three popular Ginsengs: American, Asian, and Siberian. Collectively, they are one of the ten most purchased herbs in the United States. Siberian Ginseng is not a true Ginseng, but a cousin to the other two. It is Eleutherococcus senticosus, has its own set of phytochemicals, and grows in North Eastern Europe and Asia. It is a milder tonic, great for stress and athletes, and equally beneficial for men and women. It has been extensively studied by the Soviets, and the plant for which they contrived the term "adaptogen." However, space does not allow an in-depth discussion of Siberian Ginseng at this time.

The two major species of Ginseng, Panax Ginseng and American Ginseng, are a plateful to cover all by themselves, having been part of medicine for 5000 years. American Ginseng grows wild in the rich, cool hardwood forests of the United States and Canada. Panax Ginseng grows in China, Japan, Korea, and other Asian countries.

Ginseng is a short perennial plant with three to seven compound leaves (quinquefolium has five). The root, which is the part of the plant used medicinally, differs between the two species. American root is more fibrous and looks like a beard. The Asian root has a more compact form and looks more human-shaped. The Chinese word for Ginseng, *shen-seng*, means "man root," or "like a man," because of this human shape, and supports its reputation of strengthening any part of the body. Interestingly enough, the American Indian name for American Ginseng is *garantoquen*, which has the same meaning. The Greek word "Panax," refers to a goddess believed to be a "heal all."

The roots of Ginseng are processed in two manners. One way is to peel and sun-dry the root. This is called White Ginseng. The other method is to steam the unpeeled root and dry it. This is Red Ginseng. Once the roots are processed, they are usually chopped, powdered, or extracted.

It takes six or seven years for a Ginseng root to achieve the weight necessary to support a high enough level of active ingredients. The older the root, the greater the value. This makes Ginseng a major target for foul play. To stretch Ginseng production, sometimes younger roots, inactive or unrelated plant material are added into the final product. To disguise the lack or actives, Ginseng aerial portions of the plant are added in to artificially drive up the ginsenoside level. The problem with this is two-fold. Adding plant tops throws off the ratio of these glycosides, and the above ground portion part of the plant carries toxicity.

Chinese emperor Shen Nung (3000 BC) recommended the herb for "enlightening the mind, increasing the wisdom and longevity." Not much has changed in 5000 years; Ginseng is still Asian medicine's key ingredient for revitalizing one's inner life force that they call Chi (qi). Ginseng was brought to Europeans by Marco Polo. Father Petrus Jartoux, a Jesuit missionary, introduced Asian Ginseng to the West in the early 1700s. And, in turn, due to the enormous demand for Ginseng in China, the Jesuits of Canada began exporting American Ginseng to the Orient in 1718, yielding enormous profits. This practice is still active today.

Native Americans used Ginseng for pain during childbirth, to increase fertility, to treat shortness of breath, for nosebleed, upset stomach, and female problems. Even Daniel Boone got in on the Ginseng rush. He personally collected large amounts of the root and purchased more from white settlers. In the winter of 1787, he headed up the Ohio River with 15 tons of Ginseng. Had he not managed to overturn the boat, he would have made himself a few bucks. Unruffled, the following year, he collected himself another 15 tons.

Until 1882, Ginseng was considered a useful stimulant and appetite enhancer by mainstream medicine, and was monographed in the *United States Pharmacopoeia*. It is still listed in the national pharmacopoeias of Austria, China, France, German, Japan, Switzerland, and Russia.

Science:

Ginseng contains various actives, the primary ones being saponin glycosides called ginsenosides (or panaxosides). Over two dozen ginsenosides have been isolated and catalogued. They are differentiated by a capital letter 'R" followed by a subscript number and or letter, e.g. Ra, or Rb-1). Rg1 and Rb1 are two major Ginseng factors. The two are therapeutically diametrically opposed to each other, and the ratio in which they are present will affect the pharmacology of the plant.

Asian Ginseng is much richer in Rg1 than Rb1. American Ginseng is richer in Rb1 than Rg1. Some of the Rb1 fraction (American Ginseng) properties are:

➢ Alcohol soluble
➢ Anticonvulsant
➢ Analgesic
➢ Antipsychotic
➢ Central nervous system relaxing
➢ Hypotensive
➢ GI protectant
➢ Accelerates glycolysis
➢ Increases RNA synthesis
➢ *Yin* enhancer (feminine) – Cooling, relaxing, and soothing while giving energy to the body and mind. Reduces heat of the respiratory or digestive system.

Some of the Rg1 fraction (Asian Ginseng) properties are:

> ➤ Central nervous system stimulating
> ➤ Activates brain activity
> ➤ Hypertensive
> ➤ Anti-fatigue
> ➤ Regulates blood sugar
> ➤ Up-regulates mental acuity
> ➤ Anabolic
> ➤ Yang enhancer (male) – Warming while stimulating the mind and body. A heat raising tonic for the blood and circulatory system.

Both Ginsengs make great tonics, but the ratio of Rg1 to Rb1 give them different personalities, so they can be used for different patient profiles. This tonic effect is also referred to by a Russian term, adaptogen. Adaptogens are substances that assist the body during physical, biological, or chemical stress, ennabling it to regulate itself and regain its equilibrium. The net result is an increase in vitality and physical wellness.

Using the large paintbrush of generalization and making broad strokes, one can say that Asian Ginseng is not for females, people with high blood pressure, or for long term use. American Ginseng is used by males and females alike, is safe for people with high blood pressure, and can be used for extended periods, but does not give the energy lift Asian Ginseng does. Having said all that, there are probably so many exceptions to the rules that you might as well not have the rules.

American Ginseng relaxes the brain, while having a lifting effect on vital organs. It relieves fatigue by giving energy but has an underlying calming effect. It helps lower blood pressure, fights fever, reduces inflammation, lowers cholesterol, and can be used during cold or flu (because it is cooling). Asian Ginseng acts on the pituitary to simulate the adrenals. It heightens nerve reflexes, enhances mental function, and fights fatigue. It strengthens cardiac output, hence possibly up-regulating blood pressure. It tones the lungs, stimulates sexual func-tion (in both men and women), and reduces blood sugar. It also lowers cholesterol, but also increases protein synthesis as well as appetite. Because it is heating, it should not be used during a cold and flu.

The following represents actions of Ginseng supported by human studies. Many of the mechanisms of action of Ginseng remain unclear but are based on thousands of years of use.

Stress, energy, and brain function
There is a structural similarity between ginsenosides and hormones like testosterone, estrogen, corticoids, and ACTH. Ginseng may work on the pituitary to up-regulate the body's production of stress hormones.

Ginseng may also improve the performance of athletes by increasing the uptake of oxygen by muscle. Recovery time was also shortened.

Reproductive function
Ginseng is legendary when it comes to male performance. And, studies show Ginseng increases testosterone and LH plasma levels. Ginseng has also been linked to the release of nitric oxide by endothelial cells, resulting in vasodilatation. This enhanced nitric oxide synthesis may contribute to its sexual enhancing effects. Other studies support improved penile function, libido, and participant satisfaction. What's not to be satisfied with all that good stuff?

Cardiovascular function
Ginseng can decrease cholesterol levels. The mechanisms may be a stimulation of cholesterol transport or a stimulation of cholesterol metabolism. It appears to increase HDL and prevent the oxidation of LDL.

Ginseng has demonstrated antiarrhythmic effects and has been shown to inhibit calcium channels and calcium uptake by blood vessel smooth muscle. This may explain Ginseng's hypotensive effect. The same mechanism that contributes to Ginseng's sexual effects, namely nitric oxide synthesis, also contributes to systemic vasorelaxation.

Blood sugar function
Not only Ginseng's ginsenosides, but its polysaccharides are involved in its hypoglycemic activity. While preliminary, studies show Ginseng promotes insulin release, increases receptors, and decreases receptor sensitivity.

Anticancer function
Ginseng is said to help prevent various cancers depending on the type of Ginseng, the age of the root, and the dose. American Ginseng has been shown to enhance the actions of chemotherapeutics in the treatment of breast cancer.

Immune function
Ginseng has been found to induce interferon production in addition to natural killer cell activity, and to increase phagocytosis. It has also been shown to enhance the effects of influenza vaccine and to stimulate immune function in chronic fatigue syndrome patients and patients with AIDS.

_Modern Day Uses:

Based on its adaptogenic properties, Ginseng have been used in a variety of situations covering most body systems. It has been used for:

> - Learning enhancement
> - Stress reduction
> - Fatigue reduction
> - Cardiovascular influences
> - Nervous system influences
> - Reproductive system influences
> - Endocrine and metabolic activity
> - Anti-cancer activity
> - Immunostimulatory activity
> - Drug and alcohol withdrawal
> - Radiation protectant (including passive and medical treatment)

Ginseng may be used for the following:

> Stimulant – for tiredness and exhaustion, to help with heavy tasks, examinations, long-distance driving, stage performance, athletic events, strenuous physical work, hangovers.

> Tonic – for a long-term restorative, convalescence for disease, long term fatigue, improved resistance, general free radical fighter.

> Mental benefits – improving the mental state of the elderly, depression, insomnia, mood elevator, memory, concentration, alertness, and improved learning ability.

> Stress – to cope with the strains and pains of life, protect the body from the secondary physiological effects of stress, improve defenses.

> Blood pressure – to help control high blood pressure (American Ginseng).

> Diabetes – improve blood sugar control.

> Sexual function – aphrodisiac, restore sexual function by increasing general vitality, support sex glands, increase virility, enhance male fertility.

> Menopause – improve hormone regulation, to offset the debilitating of menopause if started during peri-menopause.

> Gerontology – offset the vulnerability of the aged to stress-related conditions such as: getting cold easily, fatigue, sluggishness, a lowering of metabolic rate and the rate at which toxins are removed, as a restorative, to maintain a stable and harmonious internal state, to slow the decline of mental abilities, to improve mood, concentration, memory, and the ability to solve problems.

Dose:

Ginseng extracts should be standardized to up to 8% ginsenosides. This is about as much ginsenosides as can be concentrated out of the root without adulterating it. That is not to say that better extraction methods may one day be developed. With a high quality extract, only 100mg once or twice daily is an adequate dose.

If you prefer a high quality whole root product, take up to 6g daily in divided doses. However, remember that everybody's response to Ginseng may not be the same. Additionally, the quality of root will also be a determining factor. It is best to begin with lower doses and increase gradually.

Cautions:

Ginseng is generally well tolerated, and there are few adverse effects associated with it. For those overly sensitive, or at high doses, over stimulation and GI upset are possible. There have also been some reports by women using Ginseng long-term for PMS experiencing breast tenderness.

People with uncontrolled high blood pressure should use Panax Ginseng with caution. However, based on a 1998 study of the use of Asian Ginseng on patients with hypertension, being overly cautious may be passé. The study revealed that the Ginseng actually mildly lowered blood pressure. I still think monitoring oneself closely is a good idea until more studies confirm this outcome.

Because Ginseng has a hypoglycemic effect, diabetics should monitor their blood sugar more closely. A dosage adjustment may be necessary.

Although clinical significance is yet to be established, taking Ginseng with MAO inhibitors should be done only with the blessing of you health care professional.

References:

See General Resources

Bahrke, M, et al. "Evaluation of the Ergogenic Properties of Ginseng." *Sports Medicine.* 1994; 18:229-248

Banerjee, U, et al. "Anti-Stress and Anti-Fatigue Properties of Panax Ginseng: Comparison with Piracetam." *Acta Physiol Lat Am.* 1982; 32:277-85

Bensky, D, et al. *Chinese Herbal Medicine: Materia Medica.* Seattle, WA. Eastland Press. 1993

Chen, X. "Cardiovascular Protection by Ginsenosides and Their Nitric Oxide Releasing Action." *Clin Exp Pharmacol Physiol.* 1996; 23:728-32

Choi, H, et al. "Clinical Efficacy of Korean Ginseng for Erectile Dysfunction." *Int J Imot Res.* 1995; 7:181-6

Fulder, S. *The Ginseng Book.* Garden City Park, NY. Avery Publishing Group. 1996

Gillis, N. "Panax Ginseng Pharmacology: A Nitric Oxide Link?" *Biochem Pharmacol.* 1997; 54:1-8

Hamilton, W, et al. "Ginseng. Fact versus Myth." *Pharmacist.* 1999; 7:50-67

Han, K, et al. "Effect of Red Ginseng on Blood Pressure in Patients with Essential Hypertension and White Coat Hypertension." *Am J Chin Med.* 1998; 26:199-209

Hsu, H, et al. *Oriental Materia Medica: A Concise Guide.* Long Beach, CA. Oriental Healing Art Institute. 1986

Huang, K. *The Pharmacology of Chinese Herbs.* Boca Raton, FL. CRC Press. 1999

Le Gal, M, et al. "Pharmaton Capsules in the Treatment of Functual Fatigue: A Double Blind Study Versus Placebo Evaluated By a New Methodology." *Phytother Res.* 1996; 10:49-53

Li, J, et al. " Panax Quinquefolium Saponins Protect Low Density Lipoproteins From Oxidation." *Life Sci.* 1999; 64:53-62

Liberti, L, et al. "Evaluation of Commercial Ginseng Products." *J Pharm Sci.* 1978; 67:1487-89

Pieralisi, G, et al. "Effects of a Standardized Ginseng Extract Combined with DMEA Bitartrate, Vitamins, Minerals, and Trace Elements on Physical Performance During Exercise." *Clin Ther.* 1991; 13:373-382

Salvati, G. et al. "Effects of Panax Ginseng C.A. Meyer Saponins on Male Fertility." *Panmineva Med.* 1996; 38:249-54

Scaglione F, et al. "Efficacy and Safety of the Standardized Ginseng Extract G115 for Potentiation Vaccination against Common Cold and/of Influenza Syndrome." *Drugs Ex Clin Res*. 1997; 22: 65-72

See, D, et al. "*In Vitro* Effects of Echinacea and Ginseng on Natural Killer and Antibody Dependent Cell Cytotoxicity in Healthy Subject and Chronic Fatigue Syndrome or Acquired Immunodeficiency Syndrome Patients." *Immunopharmacology*. 1997; 35:229-235

Sotaniemi, E, et al. "Ginseng Therapy in Non-Insulin Dependent Diabetic Patients." *Diabetes Care*. 1995; 18:1373-75

Tode, T, et al. "Effect of Korean Red Ginseng on Psychological Functions in Patients with Severe Climacteric Syndromes." *Int J Gynaecol Obstet*. 1999; 67:169-74

Vuksan, V, et al. "American Ginseng Reduces Postprandial Glycemia in Nondiabetic Subjects and Subjects with Type 2 Diabetes Mellitus." *Arch Intern Med*. 2000; 160:1009-13

Yun, T. "Experimental and Epidemiological Evidence of the Cancer Preventive Effects of Panax Ginseng C. A. Meyer." *Nutrition Review*. 1996. 54:S72-S81

Yun, T, et al. "Non-Organ Specific Cancer Prevention of Ginseng: A Prospective Study in Korea." *Int J Epidemiol*. 1998; 27:359-64

Zhu, Y. *Chinese Materia Medica*. Amsterdam, Netherlands. Harwood Academic Publishers. 1998

Goldenseal

(Hydrastis canadensis)

Other Common Names:

Eye Balm, Eye Root, Goldsiegel, Ground Raspberry, Indian Dye, Indian Turmeric, Jaundice Root, Yellow Paint, Yellow Puccoon, Yellow Root, Orange Root, Wild Curcuma, Warnera, Sceau d'or

Background:

From our own Cherokee Indians

Goldenseal is a Native American plant introduced to us by the Cherokee nation from their traditional Indian medicine. The Cherokee were a friendly people who originally lived in the Tennessee River Valley. They were an ally of Andrew Jackson against the British, and during the Civil War, fought with the South. They were considered to be one of the most progressive and gifted of Indian tribes.

Goldenseal was one of the Cherokee's foremost herbs. The part of the plant used is the underground portion, called a rhizome or the root. They used it as a wash for sore mouth and inflamed eyes, a diuretic, a stimulant, and as a bitter tonic for stomach and liver disorders. They also used it for skin maladies, to treat arrow wounds and ulcers, and as a yellow dye, as the name may imply, for garments and their faces. They also mixed the root with grease to concoct an insect repellant. The first medical reference to Goldenseal was in Barton's *Vegetable Materia Medica* of 1798, when it was mentioned for the Cherokee uses of the medicine.

Professor King of the Eclectic school of medicine, in 1852, thoroughly investigated Goldenseal. He did this with many Native American plants, separating the real from the ridiculous, and brought to the medical community the positive benefits of Goldenseal, especially its use for gonorrhea and urinary tract infections. Because of his work, physicians began to demand the herb, and it became an official drug in the *U.S. Pharmacopoeia* in 1860 and stayed there until 1926.

One of the top selling herbs in the country

Goldenseal has become one of the top selling herbs in the U.S. market. But, unlike other top selling herbs that have created their groundswell of use because of overwhelming scientific validation, Goldenseal has coasted along on its folklore, that and its misguided use for blocking illicit drug testing. In fact, there hasn't been significant scientific research reported on Goldenseal since 1950, when Shideman, et al, published a major review.

Goldenseal's popularity has increased to such a level that supply shortages and a scarcity of previously wildcrafted plants has ensued. This prompted it to be nominated for a "CITES" listing. CITES stands for Convention of International Trade in Endangered Species of Wild Fauna and Flora. Over 160 countries got together and established a permit system to control trade in endangered species. Goldenseal now has an appendix I rating. That means that its trade must be monitored to avoid use incompatible with its survival.

Folkloric uses

The impressive list of historical uses that have contributed to Goldenseal's lasting popularity include:

- ➢ Antibacterial
- ➢ Antiviral
- ➢ Colds
- ➢ Respiratory congestive problems
- ➢ Bladder, vaginal, and rectal inflammations
- ➢ Inflammation of the GI, especially with respect to mucosal membranes
- ➢ Peptic ulcers, diarrhea, flatulence, gastritis, and upset stomach
- ➢ Liver and gall bladder disorders
- ➢ Topically for skin infections, impetigo, eczema, and eye inflammations
- ➢ Douche for candida
- ➢ Sedative
- ➢ Hypertension
- ➢ Menstruation difficulties
- ➢ Cancer

Science:

Hydrastine and berberine

Whatever activity Goldenseal has can be attributed to its alkaloid content, specifically hydrastine (up to 4%) and berberine (up to 6%), and to a lesser extent, other alkaloids like canadine (up to 1%). While these alkaloids are present in other plants, Goldenseal has higher levels than any other. Whereas the plant, itself, has not been the focus of clinical studies and medical documentation, for some 50 years, hydrastine and berberine, two actives in Goldenseal, have been the focus of scientific studies.

Berberine has been shown to enhance bile secretion, bilirubin, and help normalize markers in individuals with cirrhosis. It has also been shown to have anti-tumor properties, increase blood flow in the heart, and have antihistamine activity. In support of Goldenseal's popular use, berberine shows effective antibacterial activity against a long list of bacteria. It has also been effective against infectious diarrhea, including diarrhea caused by Giardia, Salmonella, and Shigella. Berberine is also shown to be an activator of macrophages, potentiating the body's ability to destroy bacteria, viruses, fungi, and tumor cells (it also interferes with the uptake of glucose into tumor cells).

Hydrastine at low doses seems be hypotensive. It has been shown to possess, as berberine, astringent and antiseptic properties. It and other Goldenseal alkaloids have been shown to inhibit muscular contractions in smooth muscle and to have an oxytocic effect (among other things, shutting down uterine bleeding).

Can Goldenseal outsmart a drug test?

There is a notion that Goldenseal will mask the results of testing for illicit drugs. This myth was born out of the writing of a famous herbal pharmacist, Dr. John Lloyd, in his 1900 novel, *Stringtown on the Pike*. The main character of this murder mystery was accused of poisoning someone with strychnine. During the trial, an expert witness testified that strychnine was present in the stomach based on alkaloid color reagent tests. A conviction ensued.

However, the heroine of the story then proves that the test for strychnine is not valid in that the same positive can be achieved by combining morphine and Goldenseal. She then presents the fact that the victim had a habit of drinking bitters with Goldenseal. The book didn't exactly have a happy ending. The main character dies in a shootout, and the expert witness commits suicide.

What the book did achieve was to provide Lloyd with his best seller out of eight books. Soon after publication of the book, expert chemical witnesses became commonplace in the American judicial system. And, attempts to use Goldenseal to dupe drug tests became the rage. It didn't take long for veterinarians to attempt to mask the use of morphine on racehorses by adding Goldenseal to their feed.

There is no scientific evidence that Goldenseal will mask the results of tests for illicit drugs.

Modern Day Uses:

It appears that the historical uses of Goldenseal, namely in cases of gastrointestinal, respiratory, and genitourinary infections, will have to be demonstrated by scientific investigations into the properties of its individual major components, like berberine. The indications for which herbalists and other alternative practitioners have prescribed Goldenseal seem to match up with the laboratory validation of its individual alkaloids.

In general terms, Goldenseal may be effective for fighting infection and for wide-ranging inflammation of the mucous membranes. The *British Herbal Compendium* notes the following indications: menorrhagia (excessively prolonged or profuse menses), atonic dyspepsia (upset stomach due to impaired tone in the muscular walls of the stomach), gastritis, mucosal inflammations, and topically in eye baths. More liberal modern uses of Goldenseal would include the following:

- ➤ Anorexia
- ➤ Antibiotic (general)
- ➤ Antiseptic (topically for burns, gum disease, mouth sores, sore throat, wounds)
- ➤ Bronchitis
- ➤ Cancer

> Colds, Coughs, Earaches, Fever, Flu
> Colon inflammation (colitis, Crohn's Disease, etc.)
> Diarrhea (infectious)
> Digestive problems
> Eye wash
> Gallbladder/Liver problems
> Gastritis
> Hepatitis
> Kidney and bladder infections
> Menstrual problems
> Swollen glands
> Skin problems topically (burns, psoriasis, eczema, ringworm)
> Tinnitus
> Vaginitis

As with any attempt to self heal, keep in mind that not all ailments are self-diagnosable and self-limiting. In many cases, professional intervention may be appropriate.

Dose:

Goldenseal oral preparations are found in a variety of forms. The most sophisticated forms are the standardized extracts. They are standardized to the total alkaloids and should come in at about 10%-12% as berberine, hydrastine and canadine. Goldenseal is many times combined with its powerful immune enhancing partner, Echinacea. When using a high powered concentrate like this, it is not necessary to take large doses.

For example when I feel myself coming down with a cold, I often use a product that contains 150 mg of standardized Goldenseal and 300 mg of standardized Echinacea. I take two tablets three times daily for two days, followed by one tablet three times daily for five to seven more days. This is generally enough time to overcome whatever was after me.

More typical dosage forms include capsulated dried root or rhizome, or tea, which can be prepared by emptying a couple of capsules into six ounces of boiling water and steeping for 10 minutes before straining. The dose of either form should be 500 mg to 1000 mg three times daily.

A mouthwash can be prepared by steeping two teaspoons full of dried plant in six ounces of boiling water for 10 minutes and straining. This can also be used as a poultice.

Cautions:

Goldenseal is generally considered to be non-toxic. However, if taken for too long or in excessive doses, its alkaloid constituents are potentially toxic and should be avoided. Symptoms of Goldenseal poisoning include GI upset, nervous symptoms, depression, and lowered heart rate. At high doses, Goldenseal can be paralyzing to the central nervous system. Prolonged use of Goldenseal may also decrease absorption of B vitamins.

This sounds very alarming but realistically, within the recommended doses, nobody should experience toxicity. Additionally, most health care professionals usually don't prescribe Goldenseal for more than a week or two at a time. Personally, if I do not see an acute condition resolved in that period of time, I generally switch to another course of action.

Because Goldenseal can stimulate uterine contractions, it should not be used during pregnancy. Its use during lactation should be avoided because it is unknown whether its alkaloids are excreted via breast milk. Better to be safe.

Because of the short duration of use for which Goldenseal is recommended, it seems almost unnecessary to mention possible interactions with other drugs. However, it is better to be conservative and be safe. Therefore, remember that Goldenseal has been used historically to lower high blood pressure. On the other hand, high doses of Goldenseal may increase blood pressure and cause cardiac problems. Therefore, if you are taking medication for blood pressure, for the week you are fighting your cold, monitor your blood pressure a little more closely, and don't overdose on your herb.

Although there does not appear to be scientific backup for the use of acidophilus (pro-biotic flora) to restore healthy intestinal bacteria, some health care professionals prescribe it during Goldenseal use. It certainly could do no harm.

References:
See General Resources

Bergner, P. "Goldenseal and the Common Cold: The Antibiotic Myth." *Medical Herbalism*. 1996-97; 8/4:1,4-6

Bolyard, J. *Medicinal Plants and Home Remedies of Appalachia*. Springfield, IL. Charles C. Thomas. 1981

Bradley, P. *British Herbal Compendium Vol. 1*. England. British Herbal Medicine Association. 1992

Bruneton, J. *Pharmacognosy, Phytochemistry, Medicinal Plants*. New York. Lavoisier. 1995

Duke, J. *Handbook of Medicinal Herbs*. Boca Raton, FL. CRC Press. 1985

Foster, S. "Masking of Drug Tests-From Fiction to Fallacy: An Historical Anomaly." *HerbalGram*. 21: 7, 35

Kumazawa, Y, et al. "Activation of Peritoneal Macrophages by Berberine-Type Alkaloids in Terms of Induction of Cytostatic Activity." *Int J Immunopharmac*. 1984; 6:587-92

Tyler, V, et al. *Pharmacognosy 8th ed*. Philadelphia,PA. Lea & Febiger. 1981

Green Tea

(Camellia sinensis)

Other Common Names:
Tea, Chinese Tea

Background:
History
Tea has been consumed for at least five thousand years for both its refreshing and health promoting benefits. Coffee drinking Westerners are generally shocked to learn that, after water, tea is the world's most popular beverage.

Legend has it that tea owes its origin to China's King Shen Nung, who in 2700 BC, was astute enough to notice leaves or blossoms which the wind had accidentally blown into his hot water. Apparently, he was brave enough to taste the new beverage and liked the taste. This is a more pleasant legend than the Indian version.

Indian legend has it that tea is a divine creation of the Buddha. Buddhism's founder, Prince Siddhartha Gautama is said to have torn off his eyelids and thrown them to the ground because he was so angered at having fallen asleep during a pilgrimage through China. Allegedly, the eyelids took root and sprouted into tea plants with leaves in the shape of eyelids. The story goes that when the Prince chewed the leaves, his fatigue disappeared, and he was able to stay awake. Then again, without eyelids, I'm not sure that sleeping was an option.

However, at the risk of hurting someone's feelings, there is archeological evidence that our prehistoric ancestors, the *homo erectus* clan, were drinkers of boiling water and leaves. There are those who speculate that these leaves could easily have been wild tea leaves, and this would have taken place 500,000 years before all the legends.

The Chinese, during the Song Dynasty (circa 1000 AD), realized the value of tea in commerce and began its export. The Dutch and British became active traders, and contributed to establishing tea as a commodity. The British later introduced the plantation system, pioneering the cultivation and manufacture of tea in India and Ceylon. This eventually broke China's monopoly on the tea trade, and by the mid-1850s, India had become the world's largest exporter of tea.

Types of Tea

The three principle types of tea products are Black Tea, Chinese Oolong Tea, and Green Tea, and although all are produced from the same leaves, their different methods of preparation make them strikingly, and medicinally different.

To make Black Tea, the leaves are rolled and exposed to air and a fermentation process, in whichh enzymes oxidize the chemicals known as polyphenols. This results in mild and flavorful beverage and makes up nearly 80% of all tea production. In black tea, the medicinal actives are reduced to an end product of 3-10%.

If the leaves are processed to destroy about half of the polyphenols, you get Oolong Tea, which accounts for 2% of all tea production. In this case, the medicinal actives are reduced to an end product of 8-20%. As a beverage, the Oolong tea is not as smooth as black tea, but not as bitter as green tea.

Green Tea is produced with the goal of preserving the leaf polyphenols. After the leaves are picked, they are steamed to inactivate the polyphenol-degrading enzymes. This is of utmost importance because it is the polyphenols, and specifically the catechin polyphenols, which give tea its primary biological and medicinal qualities.

Where does all the green tea hype come from?

Evidence of Green Tea being a health promoter comes from studying the Japanese. They have the lowest level of heart disease and highest longevity rate of all industrialized countries. The Japanese believe that by practicing their custom of consuming large amounts of Green Tea, they can lower their risk of cancer, lower their risk of developing cardiovascular disease, control blood sugar, fight colds and flu, and prevent gum disease, cavities, and even bad breath.

A 1992 evaluation of 3,300 Japanese women practitioners of Chanoyu, a tea ceremony, suggests that their intake of Green Tea contributes to their longevity by providing a degree of protection against severe fatal diseases. Additionally, population studies have shown reduced cancer rates in central Japan, where Green Tea is produced, and people drink far higher amounts than do other Japanese. It must also be noted that Japanese men smoke more than American men but still have lower rates of lung cancer.

Science:

Polyphenols called Catechins, especially one called Epigallocatechin gallate (EGCg), are what give Green Tea its antioxidant, antimicrobial, blood thinning, and cholesterol lowering activity. Catechins are a subgroup of flavonoids found in many fruits, vegetables, and wine. EGCg is considered the most potent catechin, and many studies have been done with this isolate, but other Catechins include epicatechin gallate, epicatechin and epigallocatechin.

Catechins against cancer

Specific mechanisms of action for Catechins are numerous and complicated. They are believed to prevent cancer by neutralizing carcinogens like nitrosamines and aflatoxin. This prevents free radical damage of nucleic acids in our cells, thwarting mutations. They also protect against free radical causing radiation and block the actual binding of cancer causing agents to DNA. Catechins have also been shown to increase detoxifying liver enzymes, making carcinogens more excretable.

Research suggests other possible anticancer mechanisms. Green Tea Catechins may selectively block P-450 enzymes that begin the process of detoxifying chemicals in our body, but in the process generate carcinogenic metabolites. They also may protect cells by augmenting the cell-to-cell communication that cancer causing agents inhibit. This communication blockage is thought to be an important mechanism for tumor development.

Another possible mode of action against cancer may be Catechins' ability to occupy receptor sites needed by tumor promoters. This explains why Green Tea extract can block some cancer feeding agents but not others. That is because some mechanisms are receptor dependant and some are receptor independent.

Other actions of tea polyphenols

On the cardiovascular front, Catechins lower LDL cholesterol and triglycerides, while increasing HDL levels. Potent antioxidants, they prevent the oxidation of LDL blood fats, a necessary step for plaque formation in arteries. They also naturally thin blood by inhibiting the formation of thromboxane A2, a substance necessary for the formation of blood clots and artery constriction. Catechins inhibit platelet activation factor (PAF) by this mechanism.

By interfering with thromboxane formation and hence arterial constriction, Green Tea may be of value in controlling high blood pressure. Additionally, Catechins block the actions of an enzyme secreted by the kidneys called angiotension converting enzyme (ACE). ACE inhibitors are a class of drugs very popular in modern medicine for the treatment of hypertension.

In vitro (meaning in test tubes versus in the body), Catechins have been shown to inhibit the enzyme that converts testosterone to 5-alpha-dihydrotesterone. High 5-alpha-dihydrotesterone levels are associated with prostate inflammation, prostate cancer, and male pattern baldness.

Modern Day Uses:

Cancer

> Anti-mutagenic
>> Chemicals that alter genetic material are called mutagens. It is believed that cancer can be caused by exposure to substances in our environment, at high risk jobs, or in our diets. Antimutagenic activity against many of these carcinogens has been associated with the components in Green Tea.

> Anticancer
>> Based on a vast number of studies and reviews, it appears that the consumption of Green Tea is linked to a reduced risk of many cancers. In one study on mice, it

was reported that each step in the process of conversion to malignancy was inhibited by the Green Tea polyphenols. Many studies have concluded that tea drinkers have a lower incidence of digestive tract cancers. Green Tea offers protection against skin cancers, including those caused by radiation.

Green Tea has been associated with activities against various other cancers as well. Those cancers include liver and lung cancers, smoke induced mutations in humans, pancreatic cancer, and leukemia. There is even a report on the use of Green Tea in the treatment of breast cancer.

➢ Therapeutic

Green Tea may one day be an adjunct agent in the conventional treatment of cancer. In one study, the inhibitory effects on tumor growth was enhanced by 2 ½ times when the cancer drug, doxorubicin was given in combination with Green Tea.

Cardiovascular

➢ Atherosclerosis

It has been shown that in the high dose range (greater than 10 cups daily), Green Tea has been associated with a decrease in total serum cholesterol, LDLs (low density lipoproteins) and VLDLs (very low density lipoproteins, which are even worse for you than LDLs), and triglycerides, plus an increase in protective HDLs (high density lipoproteins). This is quite a mouthful, but it is very good news.

➢ Hypertension

Animal studies suggest that Green Tea may have a positive effect on hypertension. Human studies, as of yet, have not determined such a relationship, although there does seem to be a reduced risk of stroke. I believe more data is need in this area.

Infectious Diseases

Green Tea's antimicrobial effects are well documented. It is bactericidal, virucidal, protozoacidal, and antifungal. It may be useful in the treatment of infectious diarrheal diseases. While the jury is still out on Green Tea's effectiveness on colds and flu, I make it a point to increase my intake when traveling out of the country to help prevent food poisoning and the ensuing tourista trots.

Immune Stimulator

Green Tea appears to stimulate proliferation of certain immune system cells including Beta cells, but not T cells. This information is based on laboratory tests and has not yet been confirmed in human studies.

Longevity

Green Tea's reputation of contributing to a long disease-free life is probably based on the fact that its primary components are potent antioxidants. Since free radicals can seriously damage cells and degenerate organs, antioxidants that scavenge for them make a significant and positive contribution to wellness and longevity. In some areas of activity, Green Tea Catechins are even more potent than Vitamins E or C.

Dental Health

Green Tea is especially effective against oral bacteria. This makes it an effective agent in combating bad breath, tooth decay and gum disease. Because Catechins can be detected in human saliva up to one hour after rinsing with tea, I encourage people to substitute it for coffee after meals and swish and swallow.

Weight Control

Green Tea has thermogenic properties and promotes fat oxidation. In one human study, metabolic rate was increased 266 calories per day over the placebo group after treating with Green Tea extract. This indicates that Green Tea may be useful in the control of body composition. The test material used in this study contained 90mg of EGCg and was given three times daily.

BHP

Since Catechins selectively inhibit 5-alpha-dihydrotesterone, it is conceivable that Green Tea would make a valuable companion to Saw Palmetto and Pygeum in the treatment of benign prostate hyperplasia.

Dose:

For consumers interested in supplementing their diet with Green Tea, two options exist, either drinking brewed tea or taking a high powered dried extract concentrate in the form of a tablet. The disadvantage to consuming the tea as a beverage is that the protective effects of Green Tea intake are in the 10-20 cup per day range.

Clinical quality powdered extracts are produced by concentrating 2,000 pounds of fresh leaves to 50 pounds of dried leaves and converting that to one pound of pure extract. This yields a product that can deliver a minimum of 60% Catechin polyphenols and more importantly, almost 30% EGCg by weight. This means that just one or two tablets, or approximately 60-120mg of Catechin polyphenols, gives you the equivalent of 10-20 brewed cups of tea. However, since not all extracts are produced by this method, look on the label to verify what you are buying.

Cautions:

Since Green Tea is a food compound, it is considered a safe supplement. Based on the literature, there does not appear to be any significant side effects or toxicity associated with green tea consumption. If there were a drawback to its use, it would be the methylxanthine content. The most abundant methylxanthine in tea is caffeine. On the average, a cup of Green Tea contains 50 mg of caffeine. This is not so bad, considering that the average cup of coffee contains 150 mg of caffeine.

As with any caffeine beverage, however, over consumption by sensitive individuals results in an array of effects including, insomnia, restlessness, nervousness, irregular heart beats, diuresis, and agitation. I personally drink one or two cups of tea daily, but also supplement with a Green Tea extract that contains 8% caffeine. Each tablet is 120mg and I take two daily, giving me an additional 20 mg of caffeine.

I do not find this to be a problem.

Drinking tea has been said to promote the formation of kidney stones. This is based on the theory that caffeine induces calcium secretion, and tea contains oxalate. Most stones are made up of calcium oxalate, hence the association. However, in the real world, there have not been any reported cases of kidney stone formation attributed to Green Tea consumption.

There has been a report of the impairment of iron metabolism, leading to anemia, when infants were given eight ounces of tea daily. Now why would you want to feed an infant eight ounces of tea daily? Incidentally, there was no effect on iron metabolism in older people.

Since therapeutic doses of Green Tea have been shown to inhibit platelet activation factor, hence naturally thinning the blood, make sure your physician allows for this effect if you are taking other blood thinning pharmaceuticals.

References:

See general resources

Ahmad, N, et al. "Green Tea Polyphenol Epigallactechin-3-gallate Differentially Modulates Nuclear Factor Kappa B in Cancer Cells Versus Normal Cells." *Arch Biochem Biophys*. 2000; 376:338-346

Blot, W, et al. "Tea and Cancer." *Eur J Cancer Prev*. 1996; 5:425-38

Bu Abbas, A, et al. "Stimulation of Rat Hepatic UDP-Glucuronosyl Transferase Activity Following Treatment with Green Tea." *Food Chem Tox*. 1995; 33:27-30

Beautheac, S, et al. *The Book of Tea*. Flammarion. 1992

DiGiavanni, J. "Multistage Carcinogens is in Mouse Skin." *Pharmacol Ther*. 1992; 54:63-128

Dulloo, A, et al. Efficacy of Green Tea Extract Rich in Catechin Polyphenols and Caffeine in Increasing 24-H Energy Expenditure and Fat Oxidation in Humans." *Am J Clin Nutr*. 1999; 70:1040-5

Evans, J. *Tea in China*. New York, Greenwood Press. 1992

Imai, K, et al. "Cross Sectional Study of Effects of Drinking Green Tea on Cardiovascular and Liver Diseases." *Brit Med J.* 1995; 310:693-696

Komori, A, et al. "Anticarcinogenic Activity of Green Tea Polyphenols." *Jpn J Clin Oncol.* 1993; 23:186-190

Marks, V. *Tea: Cultivation to Consumption.* Chapman & Hall. New York. 1992

Menon, L, et al. "Anti-Metastatic Activity of Curcumin and Catechin." *Cancer Lett.* 1999; 141:159-65

Merhav, H, et al. "Tea Drinking and Microcytic Anemia in Infants." *Am J Clin Nutr.* 1985; 41:1210

Sadakata, S. et al. "Mortality Among Female Practitioners of Chanyou." *Tohoju J Exp Med.* 1992; 166:475-477

Sadzuka, Y, et al. "Modulation of Cancer Chemotherapy by Green Tea." *Clin Cancer Res.* 1998; 4:153-56

Shutsung L, et al. "Selective Inhibition of Steroid 5-α-Reductase Isoenzymes by Tea Epicatechins 3-Gallate and Epigallocatechin 3-Gallate." *Biochem Biophys Res Comm.* 1995; 214:833-838

Sigler, K, et al. "Enhancement of Gap Junctional Intercellular Communication in Tumor Promoter-Treated Cells by Components of Green Tea." *Cancer Lett.* 1993; 69:15-19

Wang, Z, et al. "Interactions of Epicatechins Derived from Green Tea with Rat Hepatic Cytochrome P-450." *Drug Metab Dispos Biol. Fate Chem.* 1988; 16:98-103

Yam, T, et al. "Microbiological Activity of Whole and Fractionated Crude Extracts of Tea and Tea Components." *FEMS Microbiol let.* 1997; 152:169-74

Yen, G, et al. "Relationship between Antimutagenic Activity and Major Components of Various Teas." *Mutagenesis.* 1996; 11:37-41

Guggul

(Commiphora mukul)

Other Common Names:

Guggulipid, Guggulgum, Guggal, Gum Guggal, Gum Guggulu, Salai Tree, Indian Bedelium

Background:

Guggul is one of the most widely sold drugs in India. It has been around Indian medicine since 600 BC. Its medicinal quality actually comes from the resin of the plant that closely resembles Myrrh. In fact, it is in the same family as the Myrrh of the Bible, C. myrrha. It has long been known to lower cholesterol and triglycerides, while maintaining or improving the ratio of HDL (good cholesterol) to LDL (bad cholesterol). Additionally, it lowers serum turbidity and can prolong coagulation time.

Traditionally, it has been used for inflammatory conditions such as arthritis, rheumatism, gout, and lumbago. It has also been used in chronic endometriosis, menstrual disorders, nervous disorders, skin diseases and as an astringent in oral hygiene for sore and swollen gums. It has even been used as a weight-reducing agent in obesity.

In Tibetan medicine, Guggul is used for diseases of the skin, anemia, edema, salivation and heaviness of the stomach.

The Mukul Myrrh tree itself is native to India, growing in the rocky habitat of Rajasthan, Gujrat, and Karnatka. It is more of a spiny shrub than a tree and will grow up to about nine feet. When the bark is injured, the tree exudes a gummy oleoresin that is called *guggul gum*. That is the medicinally active stuff.

For commercial purposes, the trees are tapped for this resin, much like Maple trees are tapped for their syrup. Through a nick on the bark of the tree, the oleoresin is tapped from November through January.

Science:

Guggul for cardiovascular support

Guggul has been the subject of hundreds of studies, and the mechanisms of its effects on blood fat levels are beginning to be understood. Particularly significant is the fact that some studies have shown the ability of Guggul to not only lower serum cholesterol and triglycerides, but to also partially reverse atherosclerosis in the aorta.

Clinical studies have shown that both purified extracts of Guggul and crude Guggul gum are capable of significantly lowering cholesterol in humans. A study of 20 patients with high blood fat levels showed Guggul more effective in lowering cholesterol than Clofibrate, a synthetic cholesterol-lowering drug.

Another study of 40 obese patients found a significant lowering of cholesterol by the tenth day of Guggul administration, with further reduction by day 21. A double cross-over study of 60 obese subjects showed the same results, while a study of 25 patients with heart disease confirmed both a reduction in cholesterol and triglycerides, and surprisingly, reversed abnormalities in the electrocardiogram in 16 of the 25 patients. A long term study in New Delhi also found Guggul superior to Clofibrate.

Some of these studies have pointed out the need for long-term therapy with Guggul. For example, in one study, serum triglycerides showed a reduction, but only after two months of administration on a regular basis. However, once the triglycerides were reduced, they stayed lower for three months following the discontinuation of Guggul therapy.

The research on this remarkable remedy has been going on for decades, and it is in widespread use in much of the industrialized world as a safe and effective agent against cardiovascular disease. How about taking 500 mg of Guggul Gum for 12 weeks and lowering serum cholesterol by an average of 24% and serum triglycerides by an average of 23%? It's been done.

The chemistry of Guggul

Medicinal Guggul is prepared by dividing it into active fractions. First, it is separated using ethyl acetate to divide it into its soluble and insoluble portions. The soluble portion is kept and the insoluble discarded, as it is toxic. This is why crude preparations of Guggul are not used in medicine as they could be associated with skin and gastrointestinal untoward effects.

The soluble portion is further processed to separate out the neutral, acid and alkaline fractions. The neutral portion is where the cholesterol-lowering goodies are hidden. The acid fraction contains phytochemicals that have anti-inflammatory activity. The neutral fraction contains the plant sterols called guggulsterones. It is the guggulsterones that modulate the body's metabolism of LDL (bad cholesterol) by increasing the uptake of LDL cholesterol by the liver.

Guggulsterones have also been shown to have thyroid enhancing activity. This would further account for Guggul's ability to lower cholesterol and help explain its traditional use for weight loss.

Modern Day Uses:
Guggul can:

  - ➤ Lower elevated cholesterol
  - ➤ Lower elevated triglycerides
  - ➤ Lower VLDL (very low density lipoproteins)
  - ➤ Lower LDL (low density lipoproteins)
  - ➤ Raise HDL (high density lipoproteins)
  - ➤ Prevent atherosclerotic vascular disease development

Dose:
Guggul dosage is based on milligrams of Guggulsterones. A clinical dose is 25mg three times daily. Therefore if you had a standardized extract of 10% Guggulsterones, you would take 250mg of this extract 3 times daily.

At least one study shows that Guggul may work better when taken with Garlic. Since Garlic is such a good lipid-lowering agent in its own right, why not? The study was done with dogs and monkeys, but Garlic is still no monkey business.

Cautions:
In the many clinical trials of Guggul reported in the literature, no significant side effects were reported.

There is a phenomena know as liver dumping. This is the process by which the body gets rid of excess cholesterol by putting it temporarily into the blood, so it can be eliminated. This may cause cholesterol levels to temporarily go up before they go down. Do not be alarmed. This is a transient effect. Remember that lipid-lowering clinical trials go for months.

Guggul has been shown to have a mild effect on platelet aggregation and fibrinolytic activity. This could affect clotting times and may be important to those on anti-coagulant therapy.

References:
See General Resources

Agarwal, R, et al. "Clinical Trial of Gugulipid a New Hypolipidemic Agent of Plant Origin in Primary Hyperlipidemia." *Indian J Med Res*. 1989; 84:626-634

Bordia, A. et al. "Effect of Gum Guggul on Fibrinolytic Activity and Platelet Adhesiveness in Coronary Artery Disease." 1979; 70:992-996

Dixit, V, et al. "Hypolipidemic Activity of Guggul Resin and Garlic in Dogs and Monkeys." *Biochem Exp Biol*. 1980; 16:421

Gopal, K, et al. "Clinical Trial of Ethyl Acetate Extract of Gum Guggul in Primary Hyperlipidemia." *Assoc Physicians India*. 1986; 34:249

Kapoor, L. *CRC Handbook of Ayurvedic Medicinal Plants*. Boca Raton, FL. CRC Press. 1990

Malhotra, S. "Pharmaceutical and Clinical Studies on the Effects of Commiphora mukul (Guggulu) and Clofibrate on Certain Aspects of Lipid Metabolism." Ph.D. thesis, All India Institute of Medical Sciences. New Delhi, India. 1973

Niyanand, S, et al. "Clinical Trials with Guggulipid: A New Hypolipidemic Agent." *J Assoc Physicians India*. 1989; 37:323

Satyavati, G. " Gum Guggul – The Success Story of an Ancient Insight Leading to a Modern Discovery." *Indian J Med Res*. 1988; 87:327

Satyavati, G. "A Promising Hypolipidemic Agent from Gum Guggul." *Econ Med Plant*. 1991; 5:47-82

Singh, V, et al. "Stimulation of Low-Density Lipoprotein Receptor Activity in Liver Membrane of Guggulsterone Treated Rats." *Pharmacol Res*. 1990; 22:37

Tripathi, Y, et al. "Thyroid Stimulating Actions of Z-Guggulsterone Obtained from Commiphora Mukul." *Planta Med*. 1984; 1:78

Gymnema

(Gymnema sylvestre)

Other Common Names:
Gurmar, Gurmur, Meshashringi, Merasingi

Background:
Gymnema is a woody, climbing vine native to central and southern India. Since the 6th century BC, Indian Ayurvedic medicine has used this plant for the treatment of a condition known then as "honey urine." Thousands of years before Western science knew what diabetes was, the Indians knew both its diagnosis (excess sugar in the urine) and its treatment. The treatment was a plant called Gurmur, and as it turns out, the plant not only effectively lowers blood sugar, but also appears to help repair damage to cells in the liver, kidney and muscle.

The name Gurmar means "sugar destroyer" based on the fact that this plant has the ability to mask the taste of sugar. Its leaves have been traditionally used as an antiperiodic (a remedy that prevents the reoccurrence of a disease that tends to come back,e.g., malaria), stomachic (aids in digestion and appetite), laxative, diuretic, and cold remedy.

Science:
The phytochemicals that give Gymnema its medicinal activity have not been completely identified. The two chemicals we are aware of are Gymnemic Acid and Gurmarin Polypeptide. Other components include resins, saponins, stigmasterol, and quercitol among others.

Our understanding of the mechanisms by which Gymnema controls blood sugar are derived from findings in animal studies that elucidate the following actions. Gymnema lowers elevated blood sugar by increasing insulin production and by facilitating glucose's cellular uptake and metabolism into glycogen. It is clear that Gymnema up-regulates enzymes involved in glucose metabolism. And, that it does so only in conditions of hyperglycemia. That is, it appears to have no effect on normal blood glucose levels.

Human studies in India are finding Gymnema valuable in controlling all key parameters of diabetic treatment. It has been shown to reduce insulin requirements, reduce fasting blood sugar, control glycosylated protein levels (a long-term measure of glucose levels rather than a snapshot picture in time), and may even stimulate pancreatic islet cell regeneration.

Gymnema studies with non-insulin dependent diabetics have allowed subjects to decrease conventional drug dosages, some being able to maintain normal blood sugar levels using Gymnema alone. In insulin dependent diabetics, patients were able to reduce insulin doses with consistent improvement in blood sugar levels.

Another action uncovered is that of Gymnema's ability to lower blood fats. Researchers at Jadavpurf University in Calcutta found the leaf extract to lower serum cholesterol, LDL (low density lipoproteins), VLDL (very low density lipoproteins), and triglycerides. The exact mechanism of action is not understood, but the authors believe that Gymnema either decreases synthesis, and/or, increases the metabolism of cholesterol.

A last interesting aspect of Gymnema is its use as a diet aid. The plant does have the ability to completely mask the taste of sweet. It is purported that there is a structural similarity between an atomic arrangement of a component in the leaf and sugar. If the phytochemical gets to a receptor site before the sugar, sugar can't attach. I have tried this and it works. At this time, I am not aware of any clinical studies confirming Gymnema's use as a diet aid, but theoretically, it is feasible.

Modern Day Uses:

Gymnema shows promise in the treatment of diabetes. It may also be of value as a protectant of the cardiovascular system, based on its effects on blood lipids. And, perhaps Gymnema may one day prove to be a valuable aid in the battle of the bulge.

Dose:

The typical dose of clinical grade Gymnema is 400-600 mg daily, in divided doses, of plant material standardized to 24% Gymnemic Acid. Remember that Gymnema is a long-term botanical treatment. Plan on using it continuously for at least six months.

Cautions:

No significant sides effects are to be expected other than the obvious drop in blood sugar. If you are a diabetic and are controlled on insulin or oral hypoglycemics, do not take this lightly. Work with your health care professional if you want to include Gymnema in you anti-diabetic regimen.

References:

See General Resources

Fisheye, A, et al. "Hypolipidemic and Antiatherosclerotic Effects of Oral Gymnema Sylvestre Extract in Albino Rats Fed on a High Fat Diet." *Phytother Res*. 1994; 8:118-120

Chattopadhyay, R. "Possible Mechanism of Antihyperglycemic Effect of Gymnema Sylvestre Leaf Extract. Part 1." *Gen Pharmac*. 1998; 31:495-6

Gupta, S, et al. "Experimental Studies on Pituitary Diabetes IV. Effect of Gymnema Sylvestre and Coccinia Indica against the Hyperglycemia Response of Somatropin and Corticotrophin Hormones." *Indian J Med Res*. 1964; 52:200-207

Kapoor, L. *CRC Handbook of Ayurvedic Medicinal Plants*. Boca Raton, FL. CRC Press. 1990

McCaleb, R. "New Evidence for Ayurvedic Anti-Diabetic Plant." *HerbalGram*. 1992; #26

Persaud, S, et al. "Gymnema Sylvestre Stimulates Insulin Release *In Vitro* By Increased Membrane Permeability." *Endocrinol*. 1999; 163:207-212

Prakash, A, et al. "Effect of Feeding Gymnema Sylvestre Leaves on Blood Glucose in Beryllium Nitrate Treated Rats." *J Ethnopharmacol*. 1986; 18:143-146

Shanmugasundaram, E. et al. "Use of Gymnema Sylvestre Leaf Extract in the Control of Blood Glucose in Insulin-Dependent Diabetes Mellitus." *J Ethnopharmacol*. 1990; 30:265-279

Shanmugasundaram, E. et al. "Enzyme Changes and Glucose Utilization in Diabetic Rabbits: The Effect of Gymnema Sylvestre." *J Ethnopharmacol*. 1983; 7:205-234

Hawthorn

(Crataegus oxycantha-syn. C. laevigata; C. monogyna; C. pentagyna)

Other Common Names:
English hawthorn (oxycantha), Oneseed Hawthorn (monogyna), May, Whitethorn, Haw, Maybush, and in Chinese medicine, Chinese Hawthorn (C. Pinnatifida)

Background:
History
For an herb that has been as extensively studied as Hawthorn, one may be surprised to learn that, in the world of botanical medicine, it is kind of a new kid on the block. Although some sources date the use of Hawthorn back to Dioscorides (78 AD), the general consensus is that he was probably writing about a different genus, not known for its medicinal value. Not only that, but he had little to say about this plant other than that it was a thorny bush with astringent fruit. It must be nice to have such notoriety that one can say so little about something and be mentioned for it almost 2,000 years later.

Up until the 1890s Hawthorn was traditionally valued for its astringency, as a digestive aid, a remedy for kidney stones, and as a wine for dropsy (an old word for fluid retention). It was not until 1896 that the literature first mentions Hawthorn for its most significant medical benefit, that being cardiovascular health.

By the early 1900s, Hawthorn had become a regular in the treatment of heart disease. Parke-Davis, a major pharmaceutical company, actually marketed a Crataegus preparation because it possessed "remarkable properties as a cardiac tonic."

Nomenclature
Hawthorn is a shrub native to Europe. Its name comes from a distortion of hedgethorn because it was used in Germany to separate plots of property. Its genus name, *Crataegus* comes from the Greek word

kratos, which means hard (referring to the wood), and its species name, *oxyacantha*, is also from the Greek words *oxus* and *akantha*, meaning sharp thorn.

Hawthorn is an official medicine in western Europe, having been recognized by its regulatory agencies. It is interesting that The German Commission E has approved, for cardiac indications, only one out of the four monographs it has for Hawthorn. The approved one is that which uses only leaf and flower, and not berry. At one time, berry and berry mixtures were approved also, but in 1994, the Commissioners turned themselves around. The reason was that most of the clinical studies had been done with leaf and flower.

Science:

Preparation and Standardization

The primary actives in Hawthorn are in a class of substances called flavonoids, and specifically hyperoside, vitexin-2-rhamnoside, and oligomeric procyanidins (OPCs). The leaves of the plant are high in vitexin, and the flowers contain the most hyperoside. This is why most manufacturers often mix leaves and flowers, and berries, which contain less of both flavonoids, and probably explains why most clinical studies are done with leaf and flower.

As with many botanical medicines, the quality of various Hawthorn products can vary greatly. For example, leaves harvested in May can have .05% of a specific active, while leaves harvested in August could have .14%. It is for reasons like this that Commission E establishes guidelines for approval. In the case of Hawthorn, products must be standardized based on the flavones hyperoside, vitexin-2-rhamnoside, and OPCs. Only this way can you be sure of getting the same medicine each time you purchase it.

Cardiovascular Actions

The effects of Hawthorn on the cardiovascular system are:

> ➤ Coronary vasodilatation
> ➤ Antiarrhythmic
> ➤ Cardiotonic

> Antilipidemic
> Hypotensive

Hawthorn flavonoids possess vasodilatory action. Extracts of Hawthorn dilate blood vessels in the heart, improving its blood supply. This is achieved by a relaxation of smooth muscle components in the arteries.

Hawthorn extracts improve energy production in the heart. This enhanced metabolism results in an increase in the heart muscle's force or contraction and can calm various rhythm maladies.

Hawthorn OPCs help prevent atherosclerotic plaques formed by excessive blood fats. This action is consistent with OPCs from Grapeseed Extract and Pycnogenol, with which most of us are more familiar. OPCs may even decrease the size of existing plaques.

In addition to having a direct relaxing effect on arteries, Hawthorn flavonoids inhibit angiotensin converting enzyme (ACE). This is the enzyme that converts angiotensin I to angiotensin II, a powerful artery constrictor. When this enzyme is blocked, blood vessels become relaxed and blood pressure goes down. This is the mechanism of action behind a whole class of pharmaceutical drugs called ACE inhibitors.

Modern Day Uses:
Possible uses of Hawthorn are early stages of congestive heart failure, coronary insufficiency, angina pectoris, high blood pressure (although I recommend using it in combination with other hypotensive herbs), various arrhythmic problems (paroxysmal tachycardia), and athero-sclerosis.

Dose:
Dose depends on the type of product you have to work with. For whole plant (non-standardized) the dose can be upwards of 4000-5000 mg daily in divided doses. If you have an extract, the dose could be up to 900 mg daily. I recommend using an extract, standardized to 1.8%

vitexin-2-rhamnoside,and taking 100 mg - 250 mg three times daily.

Keep in mind that most clinical studies done on Hawthorn are of at least an eight-week duration. Hawthorn is not a fast acting medicine. It should be used for months before evaluating its benefits. Some experts recommend using it for a minimum of six months.

Cautions:

Commission E does not note any adverse side effects for Hawthorn, nor does it list any contraindications. Hawthorn use is extremely safe. However, keep in mind that Commission E also follows the New York Heart Association guidelines. It only allows for the use of Hawthorn for level 2 heart disease. That means that patients have no physical activity limitations. They are comfortable at rest, but physical activity results in fatigue, palpitations, shortness of breath, or perhaps chest pain.

I am often asked by people being treated for cardiovascular disease if it is safe to take Hawthorn with the medication they are taking. My first response is, why would you want to do that? Isn't your medicine working? If not, you had better sit down with your physician and have a chat. If it is because you want to stop taking your medicine and try diet, exercise, and herbal medicines like Hawthorn, you had really better sit down with your physician. Make sure that she or he is willing to be a participant in this lifestyle change. Cardiovascular disease is the number one killer in this country, and its treatment should not be taken lightly.

Hawthorn may have a potentiating effect on heart and blood pressure medications you are taking. This is especially true for digitalis, but I would be guarded against using Hawthorn with any medication prescribed for heart or blood pressure without the input of a qualified health professional.

References:

See General Resources

Busse, W. "Standardized Crataegus Extract Monograph." *Quart Rev Nat Med.* 1996. 189-197

Brown, DJ. *Herbal Prescriptions for Better Health*. Rocklin, CA. Prima Publishing. 1996

Ernst, E. "The Clinical Efficacy of Herbal Treatments: An Overview of Recent Systematic Reviews." *The Pharmaceutical Journal*, 1999; 262: 85-87

Leuchtgens, H. "Crataegus Special Extract WS 1442 in Cardiac Insufficiency NYHA II. A Placebo Controlled Randomized Double Blind Study." *Fortschr Med.* 1993; 111:36-8

Mowrey D, *The Scientific Validation of Herbal Medicine*. New Canaan, Connecticut. Keats Publ. 1986

Nasa, Y. et al. "Protective Effect of Crataegus Extract on the Cardiac Mechanical Dysfunction in Isolated Perfused Working Rat Heart." *Arzneim Forsch Drug Res*. 1993; 43:945-9

O'Hara, M, et al. "A Review of 12 Commonly Used Medicinal Herbs." *Arch Fam Med.* 1998; 7:523-536

Schussler, M, et al. "Mycocardial Effects of Flavonoids from Crataegus Species." *Arzneim Fkorsch Drug Res*. 1995; 45:842-5

Taskov, M. "On the Coronary and Cardiotonic Action of Crataemon." *Acta Phyhsiol Pharm.* 1977; 3:53-7

Tauchert, M. et al. "Effectiveness of the Hawthorn Extract LI 132 Compared with the ACE Inhibitor Captopril." *Munch Med.* 1994. 136:27-33

Wegrowski, J. et al. "The Effect of Procyanidolic Oligomers on the Composition of Normal and Hyper-cholesterolemic Rabbit Aortas." *Biochemical Pharmacology*.1984. 33:2491-7

Weikl, A, et al. "The Influence of Crataegus in Global Cardiac Insufficiency." *Herz Gefabe*. 1993; 11:516-24

Horny Goat Weed

(Epimedium grandiflorum)

Other Common Names:
Yin Yang Huo, Epimedium

Background:
How could you not love an herb with a name like Horny Goat Weed? I actually traveled to China to research this plant and seek it out in its natural mountain habitat. Over 40 species of Epimedium have been identified around the world and most have been used in folk medicine. Of these, over 10 can be found in China. It is a low growing plant in the same family as barberry. Yin Yang Huo is mentioned in *Shen Nung's Herbal*, a 2,000-year-old Chinese classic.

Yin Yang Huo derives its name from a northern Szechuan province where it is believed that the *yin yang*, a kind of animal, takes this drug, *huo*, to promote one hundred sexual climaxes every day. This is also a province where it might not be safe to walk alone after dark, but it didn't stop me; I was on a mission.

Epimedium has been used in both Traditional Chinese Medicine and Japanese Kampo Medicine for ailments which include: infertility, hepatitis, chronic kidney diseases, certain blood dyscrasias, the "blues", senility, low back and knee pain, menstrual irregularities, as a liver tonic, and to relieve spasms and cramps in the hands and feet. However, its real claim to fame is its traditional use as a principle aphrodisiac drug.

The principle active components of Horny Goat Weed are in its flavonoids. These phytochemicals are harvest sensitive, in that the largest flavonoid yield is achieved by harvesting the plant during its flowering period. The single compound which has been pharmacologically studied, and shown to have antihepatotoxic liver protective) and immunoregulatory activity, is Icariin. This flavonoid is used as a marker and to define plant extract quality. Good extracts are standardized to 5%-10% Ecarrin.

Science:

The scientific data available on Horny Goat Weed is a blend of East meeting West.

Endocrine system

The Chinese describe Horny Goat Weed as having a Yang strengthening effect. Yang represents masculinity, heat, fire and sun. It is believed that Horny Goat Weed inhibits monoamine oxidase in the hypothalamus, which leads to an increase in dopamine in this important endocrine, immune and metabolic regulating brain structure. Dopamine levels are key for sex drive.

As a practicing pharmacist, I can remember when the drug L-Dopa was being introduced for the treatment of Parkinson's Disease. The most memorable side effect reported by convalescent hospitals was that their little old men had started chasing their little old women around the wards.

Another mechanism that may be involved is the stimulation of cyclic AMP with actions similar to gonadotropin on gonadal function, resulting in increased testosterone.

Sexual Function/Aphrodisiac

Horny Goat Weed is reported to have peripheral vasodilating effects that lead to engorgement of the penis. It can prevent impotence induced by the stress hormone cortisol, stimulates male accessory structures, increases sperm count, and increases testosterone levels as measured by 17-ketosteroid excretion.

Mood and brain activity

Horny Goat Weed, in specific research models, has up-regulated brain neurotransmitters from a hypofunctional state, while down-regulating excessive cholinergic activity in the parasympathetic nervous system. The net result is a mood and energy stimulating effect that the Chinese refer to as a Yang restorative. This is the real reason I went to China...right.

It also appears that Horny Goat Weed has an acetylcholinesterase inhibiting action. This would explain the positive effect it may have on senile dementia and senile memory loss. Additionally, animal studies show it improves cerebral blood flow and may block the calcium influx that occurs in neuronal cell death during Alzheimer's and other neurological degenerative diseases.

Immune enhancement
Horny Goat Weed has been reported to stimulate NK (natural killer) cell activity, macrophage function, and phagocytic activity of the reticuloendothial system, and to significantly enhance Interleukin-2 restoration, lymphocyte proliferation and spleen antibody forming cells during drug-induced immune suppression.

Kidney disease
Horny Goat Weed has been shown to improve immunologic inadequacy in chronic and end-stage renal failure patients. Interestingly enough, it was also found to have sexual restoring effects in some of the patients treated.

In pharmacological studies, Horny Goat Weed was used to treat chronic renal insufficiency and resulted in improvement in BUN and serum creatinine, plus inhibited hypertrophy of glomeruli. It also diminished glomerular capillary wall degeneration.

More
Ongoing research suggests that Horny Goat Weed may also be of benefit in the following areas:

Cardiovascular: peripheral vasodilator, lowers blood pressure, increases coronary blood flow by inhibiting vascular resistance via a calcium channel blocking effect (like some drugs do), inhibits platelet aggregation, inhibits thromboxane A2 (potent inducer of blood clots), and decreases excess capillary permeability.

Allergic and chronic inflammation: suppresses antibodies, may be of value in autoimmune diseases and chronic inflammatory states, decreases capillary permeability caused by histamine.

Respiratory: bronchitis, antitussive.

Blood and bone marrow: constituents have been shown to increase bone marrow cell output by 72% following depressed activity.

Athletics: the 2,000-year-old materia medica claims reinforcement of the muscles and bones, and modern scientific studies confirm anti-catabolic and testosterone enhancing actions.

Modern Day Uses:
We read and hear of many herbs with estrogenic effects. Horny Goat Weed is unusual in that it has testosterone-like effects. Based on scientific data and word of mouth, Horny Goat Weed is primarily being purchased to:

> ➤ Stimulate sexual activity in both men and women
> ➤ Increase sperm production
> ➤ Increase sexual desire
> ➤ Increase blood flow to the genitals
> ➤ Prevent loss of sexual function in men with atherosclerosis

I believe that as this herb becomes more popular in the Untied States, we will see Horny Goat Weed used alone, or incorporated in combination formulae, for a multitude of indications.

Dose:
Take 500mg to 1500mg daily. On those special occasions, take about 1000mg 90 minutes before planned activities.

Cautions:
Epimedium is considered nontoxic. In some people dizziness, nausea, dry mouth, or thirst may occur, although this is extremely rare. Men with prostate disease should use this herb with a little caution. If symptoms of prostatitis are exacerbated, discontinue using it.

References:
See General Resources

Cai, D, et al. "Clinical and Experimental Research of Epimedium Brevicornum in Relieving Neuroendocrine-Immunological Effect Inhibited by Exogenous Glucocorticoid." Huashan Hospital, Shanghai Medical University, Shanghai, 200040.

Chen, M, et al. "Effect of Monoamine Neurotransmitters in the Hypothalamus in a Cortisol Induced Rat Model of Yang Deficiency." *Chung His Chieh Ho Tsa Chih.* 1990; 10:292-4, 262.

Chen, X, et al. "Effect of Epimedium Sagittatum on Soluble IL-2 Receptor and IL-6 Levels in Patients Undergoing Hemodialysis." *Chung Hua Nei Ko Tsa Chih.* 1995; 34:102-4.

Cheng, Q, et al. "Effects of Epimedium Sagittatum on Immunopathology and Extracellular Matrices in Rats with Chronic Renal Insufficiency." *Chung Hua Nei Ko Tsa Chih.* 1994; 33:83-6.

Hsu, H. *Oriental Materia Medica.* New Haven, CT. Keats. 1986

Huand, K. *The Pharmacology of Chinese Herbs.* Boca Raton, FL. CRC Publishing,. 1999

Iinuma, M, et al. "Phagocytic Activity of Leaves of Epimedium Species on Mouse Reticuloendotherial System." *Yakugaku Zasshi.* 1990; 110:179-85.

Kuang, A, et al. "Effect of Yang Restoring Herb Medicines on the Levels of Plasma Corticosterone, Testosterone, and Triiodothyronine." *Chung His I Chieh Ho Tsa Chih.* 1989; 9:737-8,710.

Li, S, et al. "Immunopharmacology and Toxicology of the Plant Flavonoid Baojuoside-1 in Mice." *Int J Immunopharmacol.* 1994; 16:227-31.

Liang, H, et al. "Isolation and Immunomodulatory Effect of Flavonol Glycosides from Epimedium Hunanense." *Planta Med.* 1997; 63:316-9.

Liao, H et al. "Effect of Epimedium Sagittatum on Quality of Life and Cellular Immunity in Patients of Hemodialysis Maintenance." *Journal of Chinese Herb Institute.* 1991; 4:29.

Liu, C, et al. "Effects of Flavonols and Epimedium Icarine on Rabbit's Cerebral Blood Flow and Rat's Anoxemia." Department of Pharmacy, Shenyang Pharmaceutical University, Shenyang 110015.

Liu, F, et al. "Effects of Epimedium Sagittatum Maxim. Polysaccharides on DNA Synthesis of Bone Marrow Cells of "Yang Deficiency" Animal Model Caused by Hydroxyurea." *Chung Kuo Chung Yao Tsa Chih.* 1991; 16:620-2.

Liu, Z, et al. "Effect of Improving Memory and Inhibiting Acetylcholinesterase Activity by Invigorating Qi and Warming Yang Recipe." *Chung Kuo Chung His I Chieh Ho Tsa Chih.* 1993;13:675-6,646

Shan, Y. "Effect of Flavone Glycosides of Epimedium Koreanum on Murine Fibrinolytic System and Apoplectic Mortality." *Chunk Kuo I Hsueh Ko Hsueh Yuan Hsueh Pao.* 192 14:419-23.

Shen M.D., Xiao Tong. Personal Communiqué. June, 2000.

Wang, M, et al. "Effects of Epimedium Icarine on Rabbit and Dog Vascular Smooth Muscle." Zhang Baofeng, Dept. of Phys.

Wu, Jerry. Personal Communiqué. June, 2000.

Xiong Y, et al. "The Effect of Extracts from Herba Epimedii and Semen Cuscutae on the Function of Male Reproduction." Jiangzi Institute of Medical Sciences, Nanchang 330006.

Yi, Dong You. Personal Communiqué. June, 2000.

Zhao, Y, et al. "Studies on the Immuno Modulatory Action of Icariin." *Journal of Chinese Herbs.* 1996; 27:11

Yi, Ning-yu, et al. "The Effects of Yang Tonics and Yin Tonics on Beta-adronergic Receptor and M-cholinergic Receptor System." *Journal of Traditional Chinese Medicine.* 1989; 100:44, 620.

Zheng, J, et al. "Effects of Sichuan Herba Epimedii on the Concentration of Plasma Middle Molecular Substances and Sulfhydryl Group of "Yang Deficiency" Model Animal." *Chung Kuo Chung Yao Tsa Chih.* 1995; 20:238-9,254.

Zhu, You-Ping. *Chinese Materia Medica: Chemistry, Pharmacology, and Applications.* Amsterdam. Harwood Academic Publishers. 1998.

Horse Chestnut

(Aesculus hippocastanum)

Other Common Names:

Aescin, Chestnut, Escine, Buckeye, Spanish Chestnut

Background:

Horse Chestnut is native to Asia Minor, but today is widely distributed all over the northern hemisphere. It is commonly grown as a shade tree in Europe for its splendor and resistance to environmental pollution. On a recent trip to Turkey, I was fortunate to see them everywhere, and in full bloom—a beautiful sight.

Aesculus is the Latin name for an oak with edible acorns. God only knows how the name got applied to Horse Chestnut; the seeds are hardly edible, unlike its cousin, Sweet Chestnut. Hippocastanum, on the other hand, makes sense. *Ippos* is Greek for horse, and *castanon* is chestnut. The name is believed to come from the fact that its seeds were thought to be good for horses that were broken winded, and for cattle with coughs. Or, for the similarity of the seeds with horse eyes.

Many Aesculus species and several hybrids are native to North America, for example, the Ohio Buckeye. This species is often wrongly confused with the medicinal varieties from western Asia and Europe, mainly Poland.

In Eastern countries, Horse Chestnut seeds are treated and reduced to a meal to feed horses and farm animals. While toxic to humans, they do not seem to be poisonous to any of the cattle experimented with, within the limits they can be induced to eat. The horses and cattle are said to eat Horse Chestnuts, but the pigs won't touch them. They're not stupid. I once tasted a liquid extract of Horse Chestnut and wouldn't do it twice. It was so bitter that it took a day to get the taste out of my mouth.

The English botanist, John Gerard (1545-1612), described Horse

Chestnut in 1597, to be "good against the cough and spitting blood." In 1615, it came to France from Constantinople and quickly spread throughout Europe. Traditional uses of Horse Chestnut included treatment for rheumatism, nerve pain, venous congestion symptoms, asthma, bronchitis, and hemorrhoids. A tea of the leaves, heavily sweetened, has been used for coughs. The bark of the tree was used as an astringent, antiseptic, and was used as a substitute for cinchona (quinine) for malaria. Many of these applications made it into the 20th century, and extracts were marketed by Eli Lilly, a drug-manufacturing giant.

Science:

Many of the traditional remedies were made from leaves and bark, however their efficacy has not been adequately proven to today's standards. Today the part of the plant used in medicine is the seed. And since today's medical studies are done with seed extracts, for the purposes of this writing, I will be referring to only these extracts.

Horse Chestnut seed contains up to 13% of a complex of triterpene saponins known collectively as aescin (or escin). It also contains oils, flavonoids, proanthocyanidins, tannins, and more. The saponins, aescin, are considered the main active constituent of the seed extract and have been extensively studied.

Horse Chestnut can be classified as a venotonic, anti-edematous, and anti-inflammatory. Some of its mechanisms of action have been elucidated. Two major actions of Horse Chestnut are that it improves vascular resistance, or tones veins, and reduces capillary permeability, thus inhibiting the leakage of water and protein into adjacent tissues.

How does it work?

Prostaglandin production in venous tissue is thought to be a key to the regulation of vascular reactions. E series prostaglandins relax venous tissues, and F series prostaglandins produce contraction. Horse Chestnut stimulates the generation and release of prostaglandin $F2\alpha$. The resulting increased tone of the venous system has been shown to increase blood return to the heart.

Explained simply, as one ages and things slow down and get sluggish, the return of blood back to the heart is impaired. Remember, that once oxygen-depleted blood leaves the capillaries, there is no longer the pressure pushing on the blood to move as is the case in the arterial system. Veins depend on their own tone and major skeletal muscles to squeeze blood back to the heart. As blood circulation is slowed, venous pooling takes place, and water and protein leak out. This is chronic venous insufficiency, and its symptoms are leg swelling, pain, tiredness, itching, and a feeling of skin tension.

Glycosaminoglycan hydrolyses are enzymes involved in the break-down of substances called proteoglycans that influence capillary rigidity and pore size. The increased activity of these enzymes is associated with pathologic conditions of veins. It is believed that Horse Chestnut can stabilize the cell organelles, called lysosomes, limiting the release of these enzymes. This ultimately acts to diminish the size or number of holes in the capillary walls, thus decreasing leakage. This mechanism not only rationalizes the herb's effect on chronic venous insufficiency, but may also explain its effect on other disorders where local tissue edema is contributing to the pathological process, like inflamed joints, carpal tunnel syndrome, dysmenorrhea, sports injuries, Bell's palsy, disc pathology and other back injuries.

Horse Chestnut extract has also demonstrated strong antioxidant activity, specifically scavenging for wild oxygen molecules that cause lipid peroxidation. This activity may further contribute to the plant's venous benefits by helping to prevent cell damage due to oxidative stress. Additionally, it is theorized that the extract produces increases in ACTH and corticoids, anti-inflammatory hormones.

Does it work?
Over a hundred papers have been written on Horse Chestnut. One meta-analysis covering 13 good clinical reports on Horse Chestnut and chronic venous insufficiency concluded that the seed extract therapy was superior in all placebo-controlled studies. It was as effective as other medications, but without side effects, and equal to the use of compression therapy, the elastic support hose, which are the most often prescribed treatment. Horse Chestnut reduced edema by about 25%.

A study conducted by 800 German physicians, treating over 5,000 patients, concluded that pain, leg fatigue, swelling, itching, and the tendency towards edema, all improved or were abated. They also concluded that Horse Chestnut had a patient compliance advantage over compression therapy. Other studies support the use of the extract sighting reduced leg circumferences, reduced leg volumes, reduced ankle circumference, improved vascular tone, significant improvement in subjective patient complaints, and a positive overall physician rated efficacy rating.

Modern Day Uses:

Germany's Commission E has approved the use of Horse Chestnut seed extract for pathological conditions of the veins of the legs. This includes chronic venous insufficiency with its symptoms of swelling, itching, pain, leg cramps, heaviness, etc. It has also been indicated for varicose veins and hemorrhoids.

Based on the medical literature, Horse Chestnut could be considered in the treatment of, or as an adjunct therapy for, the following:

> - Chronic venous insufficiency
> - Varicose veins
> - Edema of the lower limbs
> - Hemorrhoids
> - Leg ulcers
> - Phlebitis
> - Nocturnal leg cramps
> - Frostbite
> - Foot and ankle swelling due to long distance plane flights-taken prophylactically
> - Disorders where local swelling contributes to the pathological process- arthritis, contusions, sprains, carpal tunnel syndrome, dysmenorrhea, sports injuries, Bell's palsy, disc pathology, prostate enlargement.

Horse Chestnut extract is also effective topically. It can be used as an ointment or gel and instituted in the treatment of:

> ➤ Symptoms of chronic venous insufficiency
> ➤ Varicose veins
> ➤ Bruising or contusions
> ➤ Wounds without broken skin
> ➤ Sports injuries
> ➤ Pain of the joints, ligaments, or tendons
> ➤ Post-surgical swelling to unbroken skin
> ➤ Hemorrhoids
> ➤ Swelling caused by oral and periodontal procedures to unbroken skin
> ➤ Lymphatic vessel insufficiency
> ➤ Skin damage- Horse Chestnut extract has been shown to absorb UV-B radiation

Dose:

All of the best medical studies are done with a seed extract standardized to triterpene glycosides called saponins and measured as aescin (or escin…same stuff). If you want to use a product with clinical foundation, choose an extract that will deliver 100 mg to 150 mg of aescin daily. Most of the trials were done with 100 mg, half taken in the morning and half taken in the evening.

Saponins sometimes tend to cause a little gastric upset, so some manufacturers have utilized delivery systems to short circuit this problem. Since liquid extract can't be "controlled released," and because of my personal experience with taste, I would stick to tablets or capsules.

It is interesting to note that Horse Chestnut's saponins have low bioavailability. In Germany, there is a registered drug of escin that can be used by injection. However, oral administration does work, as exemplified by the volumes of research done with it. It is therefore speculated that aescin is hydrolyzed by intestinal flora to active metabolites.

Horse Chestnut combines well with other herbs that improve peripheral circulation, and heal connective tissue. You might find combinations with Ginkgo, Bilberry, Butcher's Broom, Hawthorn, bioflavonoids (especially Rutin), and vitamins like C.

Oral doses of Horse Chestnut are not fast acting when taken for chronic conditions. Have patience. The clinical studies that support its use are generally done for four to eight week periods.

Cautions:

According to one study, from 1968 to 1989, about 900 million doses of one particular extract were prescribed. In that time, only 15 patients reported side effects. That is a pretty good track record for safety. In rare instances, the extract can cause occasional stomach upset.

Because of the reputation saponins have for being irritating, Horse Chestnut should not be applied to broken skin.

Horse Chestnut seeds have been reputed to be poisonous, however, some believe that they are non-toxic as long as the husk is separated before using. Regardless, I don't think anybody reading this book has any business eating Horse Chestnut seeds. Remember that pigs won't touch the stuff. Do what the pigs do.

Swollen tired legs is many times a complaint of pregnancy, likely due to having to carry an extra person around all day. However, at this time safety of the use of Horse Chestnut extract, even in the topical form, has not been established, and therefore it is best avoided. However, check with your obstetrician for any up to the minute developments.

References:

See General Resources

Bisler, H, et al. "Effects of Horse Chestnut Seed Extract on Transcappillary Filtration in Chronic Venous Insufficiency." *Dtch Med Wochenschr*. 1986; 111:1321-1329

Bombardelli, E, et al. "Review: Aesculus Hippocastanum." *Fitoterapia*. 1996; 67:483-511

Diehm, C, et al. "Medical Edema Protection - Clinical Benefit in Patients with Chronic Deep Vein Incompetence. A Placebo-Controlled Double-Bind Study." *Vasa*. 1992; 21:188-192

Diehm, C, et al. "Comparison of Leg Compression Stocking and Oral Horse Chestnut

Seed Extract Therapy in Patients with Chronic Venous Insufficiency." *Lancet*. 1996; 347:292-4

Ernst, E. the Clinical Efficacy of Herbal Treatments: An Overview of Recent Systematic Reviews. *The Pharmaceutical Journal*, 1999; 262: 85-87

Geissbuhler, S, et al. "Treatment of Chronic Venous Insufficiency with Aesculus Vein Gel." *Schweiz Zschr Ganzbeits Medizin*. 1999; 11:82-7

Greeske, K, et al. "Horse Chestnut Seed Extract – An Effective Therapy Principle in General Practice. Drug Therapy of Chronic Venous Insufficiency." *Forschr Med*. 1996; 114:196-200

Kreysel, H, et al. "A Possible Role of Lysosomal Enzymes in the Pathogenesis of Varicosis and the Reduction in their Serum Activity by Venostatin®." *Vasa*. 1983; 12:377-82

Longiave, D, et al. "The Mode of Action of Aescin on Isolated Veins: relationship with PGF2α." *Pharmacol Res Comm*. 1978; 10:145-53

Morgan, M, et al. "Aesculus Hippocastanum-Horse Chestnut." *MediHerb Professional Review*. 1998; 65:1-6

Pittler, M, et al. "Horse Chestnut Seed Extract for Chronic Venous Insufficiency: A Criteria Based Systematic Review." *Arch Dermatol*. 1998; 134:1356-60

Rehn D, et al. "Comparative Clinical Efficacy and Tolerability of Oxerutins and Horse Chestnut Extract in Patients with Chronic Venous Insufficiency." *Arzneim-Forsch Drug Res*. 1996; 46:483-7

Tsutsumi, S, et al. "Anti-inflammatory Effect of the Extract Aesculus Hippocastanum and Seed." *Shikwa-Gakutto*. 1967; 67:1324-8

Kava

(Piper methysticum)

Other Common Names:

Kava Kava, Ava, Kawa, Awa, Yava

Background:

Did you ever wonder what the people of the South Pacific did when they got home, after a hard day's work, before they were introduced to alcohol by Captain James Cook in the late 1700s? Well, neither did I, but they did have a great secret weapon against stress that is only now becoming very popular in the western world.

The secret weapon is called Kava, the dried creeping underground stems and roots of *Piper methysticum*, a large shrub in the pepper family from Melanesia, Micronesia, and Polynesia. For thousands of years, Kava extract, prepared as a drink has been used in Oceania for its calming effect, and its ability to make you more sociable. Imagine, they were actually able to get by without some of the best selling drugs in the world, like Valium®.

For centuries, Kava has been used in the South Pacific for its euphoric calming effect. It has also been used to relax muscles, heal wounds, mediate conflicts and family feuds, to treat epilepsy, sore throats, bronchitis, menstrual cramps, menopausal problems, toothaches, colds, rheumatism, and gout, and as an aphrodisiac. The great thing is that modern scientific research is bearing out the validity of these folk uses.

Captain James Cook and other early explorers

Although Captain Cook, on his voyage in the *Endeavor*, is usually credited with discovering Kava for the West, the plant was actually introduced to Europeans in the early 1600s by Dutch explorers, Jacob LeMaire and William Schouten. They got to see the preparation and ceremonial use of the Kava beverage and recorded what they saw in their journal. As you can see, they were a little put off by the preparation part, the reason for which will soon become clear. Schouten says,

"They presented also their desirable drink to our people, as a thing rare and delicate, but the sight of their brewing had quenched our thirst."

James Wilson, a later explorer of the Marquesas Islands and Tahiti in the years 1797-98, says, "the preparation is disgusting: several women each have a portion given to them to chew, or the stem and rot together, which when masticated, they spit into a bowl."

Captain Cook and his ship's artist, Sydney Parkinson, and botanist, Daniel Scholander, are rightfully credited with providing an extensive written record of Kava and its rituals. And George Forster, a botanist on Cook's second voyage, is credited with the formalizing of Kava. He prepared the proper description and assigned the name, Piper methysticum, which means intoxicating pepper. He also is the first to record the skin rash associated with heavy Kava use. He wrote, "The skin dries up and exfoliates in little scales."

Cook writes from Tahiti in September of 1773:

> The manner of brewing or preparing the liquor is as simple as it is disgusting to a European and is thus; several people take of the root or stem adjoining to the root and chew it into a kind of pulp when they spit it out into a platter or other vessel, every one into the same vessel; when a sufficient quantity is done, they mix with it a certain proportion of water and then strain the liquor through some fibrous stuff like fine shavings, and it is then fit for drinking which is always done immediately; it has a pepperish taste, rather flat and insipid and intoxicating.

It is said that the preferred designated Kava chewers were virgin women. I have often been accused of being easily confused but, if the job description reads "chewer," shouldn't the greatest concerns be sound teeth and a strong jaw?

Today, the chewing has been replaced by pounding or shredding the root. And, coconut milk is usually added to the strained mixture rather than water. But, once the beverage is consumed, the results are the same. Initially, the mouth becomes numb. This is followed by feelings of mellowness and well-being. One usually feels more sociable, and many people enjoy a heightened sense of awareness.

The ceremonies

The rituals have changed little over the centuries. The traditional ceremony consists of men sitting on the ground cross-legged, in a modified circle. The highest ranking person sits to one side, and the server sits in the center next to the Kava bowl. Things begin with the reciting of chants over the guest, the roots, and the hooch. The server ladles the drink into a cocoanut shell, and it is served in descending pecking order. The drinker guzzles the entire shell to the sounds of clapping and chants. This goes on for sometimes dozens of rounds, or until no pain is felt anywhere.

There are three major types of ceremonies. The full-blown version is enacted on very formal occasions, such as welcoming royalty or a very important guest. There is the ceremony performed at the meeting of village elders, chiefs, and nobles, or visiting chiefs and dignitaries. And there is the less formal meeting at the village watering hole.

In most Kava societies, women were not allowed to partake in the joys of root, even though they were allowed to be chewing machines. On some islands, Kava drinking was restricted to royalty and breaking the rules was punishable by death. In other cultures, like Hawaii, common folks were allowed to drink Kava for their enjoyment after a hard day's work in the jungle.

The origin of Kava

Kava has been cultivated for so many thousands of years that its exact origin is not entirely clear. The form we use today is a product of evolution. Most authoritative societies recognize at least 12 varieties of Kava. About 80 were identified on Vanuatu, a chain of volcanic islands between Australia and Fiji. Because Vanuatu is the site of Kava's greatest differentiation, it is theorized that Kava originated there. Chemical analysis of *Piper methysticum* suggests that it is a domesticated cultivar derived from *Piper wichmannii*, wild Kava. *P. wichumannii* is also indigenous to Vanuatu.

Science:

Kavalactones

Chemistry-wise Kava-Kava owes its effects to a collection of fat-soluble pyrones called kavalactones. About 15 of these have been identified, with 6 being the predominant players, but it is believed that they all work together synergistically and must all be present to induce the whole suite of psychoactive activity for which Kava-Kava has become famous. Archeologists have discovered chemical traces of these actives in Pacific Islands' antiquities that are thousands of years old.

Recent studies on comparative chemistry of various Kava plants show that different cultivars contain different mixtures of kavalactones. This can actually alter the actions of the end product. For example, if the ratio of two components goes one way, the effects can be a fast onset, relaxation, and a fresh feeling of well being. If they go the other way, the effects can be a slow onset, depressant action, and a hangover effect. Over time, the local growers have learned to culture their plants for the most desirable effects. Manufacturers have to trust where their raw material comes from. Some of the finest product originates in Vanuatu.

Kava, the psychoactive

Research on kavalactones' mechanism of action on the central nervous system is basically suggestive, and no clear consensus has been reached. Because of the similarities in action to benzodiazepine drugs (Valium® types), it has been theorized that the CNS effects may be due to potentiating receptor sites of the relaxing neurotransmitter, GABA. However, it is speculated that rather than work on the higher centers of the brain, kavalactones influence a more primitive part of the CNS responsible for emotions like fear, anger, and sadness. This area is called the limbic system.

One study I came across tested the effectiveness of Kava on normal healthy adults experiencing stress and anxiety associated with the day-to-day aggravations of living. The researchers concluded that Kava was effective and offered an alternative to benzodiazepines to reduce anxiety. I guess they figured that a "non-clinical sample of adults" turn to drugs for their daily stress. And perhaps it's true because, before commencing with the study, one of the things the researchers had to do was to ask their subjects to discontinue their anxiolytics, antidepressants, sedative and neuroleptics for a period of time equal to at lest five half-lives of their drugs. That says a lot for "normal."

Kava, the anticonvulsant, analgesic, and muscle relaxant

Kava pyrones can inhibit convulsions intentionally induced by drugs. Studies show that this activity is mediated by way of the same receptor sites targeted by anti-epileptic drugs. Kava pyrones also have an analgesic effect that we believe occurs via non-opiate pathways. Some kavalactones are said to have pain-relieving effects similar to aspirin.

Kavalactones are excellent muscle-relaxing agents. They work by depressing the magnitude muscle end plate potentials without effecting their frequency. This means that they work on muscle contractions but don't work by blocking neurotransmission. There is also a kavalactone that has a similar effect on smooth muscle by raising extracellular potassium concentrations while blocking potassium channels. This may explain its soothing action on irritable bladders.

Modern Day Uses:

In its monograph on Kava, Commission E, a division of the German equivalent of the FDA, finds Kava an acceptable therapeutic option for conditions of nervous anxiety, stress, and restlessness.

Kava-Kava's anti-anxiety activity, plus its sedative and relaxing actions are well documented around the world. It is used to soothe nerves, induce relaxation and sleep, and counteract fatigue. However, unlike modern tranquilizers, Kava Kava leaves the user with an alert mind, enhancing the ability to communicate while sharpening the senses. Unlike alcohol or other drugs, Kava provides relaxation combined with the ability to act when necessary.

Consider Kava for:

> ➢ Anxiety
> ➢ Tension

> Stress
> Restlessness
> Sleep
> Muscle relaxant
> PMS symptoms such as anger and cramps
> Menopausal systems
> Irritable bladder syndrome

Dose:

There are several good quality Kava standardized extracts available. Some are titrated to 30% kavalactones, some to 40% kavalactones, and others to 70% kavalactones. What is important is that at the end of the day, you end up with between about 140 mg to 210 mg of kavalactones.

Based on typical European studies, the effective dose of Kava, as kavalactones, is 70 mg three times daily. Studies are generally done for several weeks, but I recommend cycling Kava, discontinuing its use when life stops beating up on you and going back on it as needed.

However, I have seen positive outcome studies that were run at 120 mg twice daily. Perhaps those wishing to use Kava should experiment to see what dosing regimen works best for them. To determine the amount of actives you will get, multiply the percentage Kavalactones by the total milligrams. If you have 100mg and 70% are kavalactones, you have 70mg of kavalactones. If you have 100mg and the kavalactones are 40mg, you have 40mg.

Cautions:

Kava-Kava has been studied extensively to determine if there are any significant or long-term dangers in using it, and none have been found. One review of the safety of Kava concluded that, when used in the doses mentioned above, Kava appears to offer safe and effective anti-anxiety and muscle relaxant actions without depressing centers of higher thought.

German Commission E warns against the use of Kava during pregnancy, lactation, or in cases of endogenous depression (depression without external causes). Even though the literature boasts the heightened senses some people achieve when taking Kava, I would discourage driving or operating machinery under the influence of Kava. Under no circumstances should you try to drive under the influence of Kava if you have not experienced how your body reacts to it. Effects of Kava can be enhanced if taken with other depressant drugs or alcohol.

Alcohol can increase the effects of Kava-Kava, even though a recent study designed to prove that concluded that the two were not synergistic. But I still do not recommend concomitant use, although one of my closest colleagues has been known to sometimes end his day with a couple of capsules and a glass of wine. Mind you, that this is done at home and at bedtime.

Kava is a relaxant. It should not be used with central nervous system depressant drugs, unless prescribed so by your healthcare professional. Using concomitantly will have an additive depressant effect.

Probably the most pronounced side effect of Kava-Kava, besides rare mild gastrointestinal disturbances, is that it has been reported to be a female aphrodisiac. In moderate doses, it has been shown to markedly increase female libido. And this from a plant that is dependent on humans for its propagation because it can no longer reproduce sexually.

And as far as the dreaded skin problems Cook's crew reported in 1773, if you experience scaly or scabby skin, you're taking too much. This undesirable side effect only occurs when copious quantities are consumed for a long time.

References:
See General Resources

Anon. "Monograph: Piper Methysticum (Kava Kava)." *Alt Med Rev.* 1998; 3:458-460

Bone, K. "Kava- A Safe Herbal Treatment for Anxiety." *Brit J Phytotherapy.* 1994; 3:147-153

Emser, W, et al. "Improvement of Sleep Quality." *TW Neurology/Psychiatry*. 1991; 5:636-42

Hansel, R. "Kava-Kava in Contemporary Medical Research: Portrait of a Medicinal Plant." *European Journal of Herbal Medicine*. 1998; 3:17-23

Herberg, K. "Driving Competence After Ingestion of Kava – Special Extract WS 1490." *Z Allg Med*. 1991; 67:842-6

Lebot, V, et al. *Kava: The Pacific Drug*. New Haven, Yale University Press. 1992

Lehmann, E, et al. "Efficacy of a Special Kava Extract (*Piper Methysticum*) in Patients with States of Anxiety, Tension and Excitedness of Non-Mental Origin – A Double-Blind Placebo-controlled Study of Four Weeks Treatment" 1996; *Phytomedicine*. 3:113-19

Norton, S, et al. "Kava Dermopathy." *Journal of the American Academy of Dermatology*. 1994; 31:89-97

Piscopo, G. "Kava Kava: Gift of the Islands." *Alternative Medicine Review*. 1997; 2:355-64

Pittler, M, et al. "Efficacy of Kava Extract for Treating Anxiety; Systematic Review and Meta-Analysis." *J Psychopharmacol*. 2000; 20:84-9

Singh, Y. "Kava: An Overview." *J Ethnopharmacol*. 1992; 37:13-45

Singh, N, et al. "Randomized, Double-Blind, Placebo-Controlled Study on the Effectiveness and Safety of Kavatrol® in a Non-Clinical Sample of Adults with Daily Stress and Anxiety." Unpublished Manuscript, 1998

Woelk, H, et al. "A Comparison of Kava Special Extract WS 1490 and Benzodiazepines in Patients with Anxiety." *Z Allg Med*. 1993; 69:271-7

Kudzu

(Pueraria lobata)

Other Common Names:
Japanese Arrowroot, Ge-gen

Background:
Kudzu is considered a noxious weed in the South, covering some seven million acres of it. A coarse, high-climbing vine with a huge root, Kudzu is often the size of a human body. In fact, Kudzu is one of the world's largest vegetable roots. A member of the legume family, it has been part of Chinese and Japanese cooking for thousands of years.

Kudzu was introduced to the U.S. around the turn of the century. It promised to be the solution to soil erosion, as well as a food for grazing livestock. However, it has done a bit too well and literally has overrun millions of acres, swallowing native vegetation and everything else in its way, including buildings. If you live in the South, and Kudzu is growing towards your neighborhood, get a goat. If that doesn't work, consider napalm.

> *In Georgia, the legend says*
> *That you must close your windows*
> *At night to keep it out of the house.*
> *The glass is tinged with green, even so...*

From the poem, "Kudzu," by James Dickey

In China, Kudzu has been part of traditional Chinese medicine since around 200 BC. It has since been used by the Chinese and Japanese, in their Kampo medicine, as a treatment for something called "superficial diseases," which are problems manifested under the skin, having yet to "reach the surface." Additional uses have included, lack of perspiration, headaches, diarrhea, dysentery, skin eruptions, high blood pressure, angina pectoris, sudden deafness, to improve cerebral circulation, and as a folk remedy to "sober-up an unconscious drunk."

Science:

Kudzu root is high in isoflavones and isoflavone glycosides, the key constituents including daidzein, diadzin and puerarin. Depending on growing conditions and geographics, total isoflavones can vary from 2-12%. Puerarin is most prevalent, followed by diadzin and daidzein.

Flavonoids are generally associated with being modulators of microcirculation, improving circulation. This is the case with the components of Kudzu. Fractions of Kudzu root have been evaluated for their cardiovascular effects and found to dilate coronary and cerebral arteries, increasing blood flow. They have been shown to decrease vascular resistance, decrease oxygen consumption in heart muscle, and increase blood oxygen supply.

Additionally, Kudzu extracts also have been shown to be anti-arrhythmic, and to decrease blood pressure, heart rate and plasma renin (a hypertension culprit) activity in hypertensive test animals. Alcohol and water extracts have shown a variety of actions consistent with many of Kudzu's historical uses, and perhaps more studies will be performed, if for no other reason than to save the South from this dreaded invader. I think the only way we are going to control Kudzu is to find more uses for it and use it up.

Modern Day Uses:

While there are encouraging studies pointing to Kudzu's supportive benefits for angina pectoris and high blood pressure, a fascinating breakthrough came in a landmark and heavily publicized study released in 1993. As a result of this study, performed at Harvard Medical School, researchers Wing-Ming Keung et al. concluded that Kudzu might be helpful in reducing the urge for alcohol and as a complementary treatment for alcoholism.

Kudzu and alcoholism

In the experiment, Syrian Golden hamsters, which are bred to be drunks, were tested to see if the Kudzu would affect their free choice of beverages. Given a choice between booze and water, these hamsters will normally increase their consumption of alcohol and decrease their consumption of water to levels hazardous to their health. I am sure we all have friends known to exhibit the same behavior.

Kudzu root extract administration effectively reduced their alcohol intake and increased their water intake. This activity is believed to be the result of the reversible inhibition of enzyme alcohol dehydrogenase and aldehyde dehydrogenase by the isoflavones contained in the root. Then, to validate the Golden hamster in assessing this anti-alcohol treatment, the hamsters were tested with other anti-alcoholism drugs. "The results clearly indicate that the suppression of free-choice ethanol in the Golden hamster is completely consistent with the beneficial effects of these agents as observed in alcohol-dependent humans."

It looks as though Harvard is really on to something. Of course, not to derogate Harvard's work, the use of Kudzu as a medicine to treat alcohol-related diseases was first documented in the Chinese Pharmacopoeia of 600 AD. Clever, those Chinese.

Pour me another tequila, Sheila
My personal interest in Kudzu comes from reports of its historical use to both forfend and treat hangovers. I am sure that it is no secret to any of us that as we age, we tend to lose our "party" gene. What we used to be able to do, and tolerate the results of, in "party mode" tends to leave us. In my household, we are lovers of wine. When my wife prepares the occasional gourmet meal, we like to match our courses with fine wines. In an effort to reduce the effects of one too many tastings, we take Kudzu. We, and our dinner guests, are great advocates of using Kudzu before, during, and after consuming alcohol.

Another interesting note on Kudzu and alcohol use is that of liver protection. Before Keung conducted his research at Harvard, he traveled to China to gather information. He interviewed many physicians and reviewed 300 case studies. One of the secondary conclusions he was capable of drawing was that Kudzu was able to improve the function of alcohol-affected vital organs. This was validated at Jiwaji University in India, when their research determined that Kudzu helps stimulate regeneration of the liver and makes the liver more resistant to damage from poisons.

Dose:

The dose of Kudzu will depend on the type of product you are purchasing. For example, the 1985 Chinese Pharmacopoeia suggests 9-15 grams of root. However, in China they make a standardized product where 10 mg. is equivalent to 1.5 grams of crude root. This means the dose would be 30-120mg in two to three divided doses daily. Keep in mind that this dose is indicated for the treatment of angina pectoris.

For various preparations, it is best to follow the manufacturer's recommendations.

Cautions:

Do not drink and drive.

Kudzu is considered completely non-toxic. However, for those who are taking blood pressure or heart medications, remember that Kudzu may potentiate their effects. If you are taking blood pressure medication, discuss possible things to look for with a health care professional if you intend to use Kudzu for any length of time.

References:

See General Resources

Foster, S. "Kudzu Monograph." *Quarterly Review of Natural Medicine* Winter: 303-8.

Keung, W. and Vallee, B "Daidzein and Daidzein Suppress Free-Choice Ethanol Intake by Syrian Golden Hamsters," *Proc. Nat. Acad. Sci.* 1993; 90: 10008-12.

Shukla, S. et al. "Protective Action of Butanolic Extract of Pueraria tuberosa DC against Carbon Tetrachloride-Induced Hepatotoxicity in Adult Rats." *Phytotherapy Research* 1996 10:608-9.

The Amazing Story of Kudzu. http://www.cptr.ua.edu/kudzu/

Licorice

(Glycyrrhiza glabra)

Other Common Names:

Spanish Licorice, Russian Licorice, Turkish Licorice, European Licorice, Gancao, Sweet Root, Yasti-madhu, Glycyrrhiza

Background:

Licorice is native to the Mediterranean region but is today cultivated throughout Europe, the Middle East, and Asia. One of the most widely used medicinal herbs in Traditional Chinese Medicine (TCM), it is found in numerous traditional formulae. It may also be the best studied herb in the world.

The first account of the cultivation of Licorice comes from Italy in the 13th century. Before that, it is believed to have been only wildcrafted. Cultivated roots and rhizomes are harvested after four years of growth. Millions of pounds of licorice are imported into the United States annually. Ninety percent of these pounds go to the tobacco industry as a flavoring agent, while much of the remaining ten percent goes to food and liquor commerce. Most licorice candy in the United States is licorice-free, being flavored with anise oil. Authentic licorice candy must generally be imported from Europe.

The use of Licorice is first documented in Assyrian clay tablets (2500 BC). When Tutankhamen's tomb was opened, pieces of licorice were found in jars around his treasures. Napoleon liked to chew on it because it calmed his nerves while in battle, and then relieved his stomachache when things didn't go so well. Monks of the Middle Ages used it for chest infection and coughs. And, our Sioux Indians chewed on it to relieve toothaches and made eardrops from it to quell earaches. In 1760, a British pharmacist added sugar and flour to it and made it a candy. No, his name wasn't Good or Plenty, but Dunhill.

The Greeks were the first to mention Licorice in the 3rd century BC. Hippocrates and Theophrastus adorned its uses and commented on its sweetness, it being 50 times sweeter than sugar, and touted it for asthma, dry cough, and chest disorders. Dioscorides (1st century AD) named the plant Glyrrhiza, Greek for sweet root. And talk about having a shelf-life, sample of historic Licorice form 756 AD was analyzed and found to still have its active principles intact after 1200 years.

Science:

Licorice is metabolized and excreted from the body by the liver and appears to have an effect on every system of the body. The major active component of Licorice is a saponin-like glycoside called glycyrrhizin (also referred to as glycyrrhizic acid or glycyrrhizinic acid). Its primary metabolite is glycyrrhetic acid (also referred to as glycyrrhetinic acid). It makes up 5-10% of the root by weight depending on the growing conditions. Other actives include isoflavonoids, coumarins, tripenoids, sterols, lignins, and volatile oils.

Anti-inflammatory effects

Glycyrrhizin is similar in structure and activity to adrenal steroids. Therefore, it should come as no surprise that Licorice has anti-inflammatory activity similar to cortisone and has been found useful for arthritis and allergies. It can bind to glucocorticoid receptors, enhancing the body's cortisol activity, or potentiate drugs like prednisone. It also inactivates the enzyme that converts active cortisol to its inactive form.

Licorice is also used for mild Addison's disease and other primary adrenal insufficiencies, such as hypoglycemia. Because Licorice increases cortisol levels, and cortisol is a very strong stimulator of mineralocorticoid receptors in the kidney, licorice may, in large doses, cause sodium retention, potassium depletion, and water retention. Excess consumption may lead to classic symptoms of hypertension: edema, increased blood pressure, potassium loss, and muscular weakness.

Licorice may prove one day to be a treatment for Lupus and other autoimmune diseases, either alone, or in combination with other herbs. Japanese researchers, in search of substances that might be used against autoimmune diseases, found Licorice to increase the clearance of the autoimmune-producing excess immune complexes. The medicine was produced in the old fashioned Chinese tea-pot method of, in this case, boiling 250 gm of root in two liters of water and cooking it down to one liter.

Based on the fact that people with Chronic Fatigue Syndrome respond to drugs with strong mineralocorticoid activity, there has been some interest in Licorice as an adjunct therapy for this disease. While more research is necessary, there have been some positive outcomes reported.

Estrogenic effects
The hormonal effects of Licorice are a little complicated. At low doses, it appears to have anti-estrogenic actions and at higher doses, it will potentiate estrogen action. These activities are due to Licorice's isoflavone and sterol content.

Because of Licorice's antiestrogenic actions, and perhaps its ability to suppress progesterone degradation, it is a valuable hormone balancer prior to menses. By affecting the estrogen-progesterone ratio during the midluteal phase (two weeks prior to menstruation), it has been shown to mediate PMS symptoms.

Immune and antimicrobial effects
While other phytochemicals (flavonoids) appear to be responsible for the anti-bacterial and anti-parasitic effects of Licorice, glycyrrhizic acid seems to possess anti-viral properties. The exact mechanisms remain unclear, but it is believed that Licorice acts on the protective protein coating of the virus in addition to inducing interferon, the body's natural viral fighter.

There has been recent interest in Licorice's ability to inhibit the AIDS virus. Using Licorice fractions and proprietary compounds derived from Licorice, researchers have been able to prevent HIV patients from developing AIDS, block the progression of immunological abnormalities, increase helper T cell counts, improve helper to suppressor ratios, improve liver function, and in some cases, show a reduction or disappearance of the "p24 antigen" (a marker for active disease).

Licorice also has anti-fungal properties, having been shown to inhibit the growth of Candida albicans. Its anti-parasitic effects have led Japanese researchers to try to develop a new anti-malaria drug from Licorice.

Liver effects
Licorice has been shown to inhibit chemical assaults on the liver, thus preventing damage. It acts to prevent free radical formation. In addition, human studies have demonstrated impressive results in the treatment of hepatic failure, infectious hepatitis, and hepatitis B and C.

Gastric effects
In 1946, a Dutch pharmacist noticed that his patients with peptic ulcers were great fans of Licorice candies. When he inquired, he was told that the candy worked better than the medicine they were taking for the relief of their discomfort. The pharmacist published his account in a Dutch medical journal, and soon studies were published in journals around the world showing that Licorice extracts can heal ulcers.

Licorice works differently than standard ulcer drugs that suppress acid secretions. Licorice works by affecting two prostaglandins (short-term hormone-like substances), PGF2 and PGE2 alpha. Licorice inhibits the enzymes that convert these prostaglandins to their inactive form. When these prostaglandins stay high, the cells in the stomach lining continue to divide at a higher rate than normal, and the quality of the gastric lining improves. And, as an extra benefit, Licorice has an anti-spasmodic effect.

The great draw back to using Licorice for ulcers was the potential side effects of glycyrrhetinic acid. This problem was overcome when a deglycyrrhizinated was developed and found to be equally effective, as the antiulcer activity of Licorice must not depend on glycyrrhetinic acid, but probably its flavonoids. Today, most herbalists prefer the Deglycyrrhizinated Licorice (DGL) to the standard extracts, but only for peptic ulcer disease.

This is a bit of a mute point today. With the startling discovery that peptic ulcers are caused by the bacteria, Helicobacter pylori, antibiotic therapy has become the new primary ulcer therapy. This is not to say that DGL does not have its place in complimentary medicine. DGL can be of great value in patients on long term therapy for arthritis with ulcerogenic drugs like aspirin, other nonsteroidal anti-inflammatory drugs, or any "gut eating" chronic medication, for that matter.

Respiratory effects
In addition to the general anti-inflammatory benefits mentioned above, Licorice also has anti-tussive (cough suppressing) and expectorant (mucus thinning) activity, allowing it to be useful for asthma.

Anticancer effects
Licorice has anti-mutagenic properties. It appears to prevent cancer promoters from binding to cells.

Topical effects
Because of the anti-inflammatory, antibacterial, and antiviral effects of Licorice, topical preparations have been shown to be useful. Areas that have been given attention are: herpes simplex (both oral and genital), eczema, psoriasis, and the prevention of general wound infections.

Modern Day Uses:
When used responsibly, Licorice can be useful for:

> - Arthritis
> - Rheumatoid arthritis
> - Asthma
> - Addison's Disease
> - Adrenal insufficiency
> - PMS
> - Menopause
> - Colds, Flu, Cough
> - Liver disease
> - AIDS
> - Peptic ulcer disease

➤ Gastritis
➤ Lupus
➤ Hypoglycemia
➤ Bronchitis

Licorice preparations for the skin can be useful for:

➤ Herpes
➤ Eczema
➤ Psoriasis
➤ Prevention of wound infections
➤ Various types of dermatitis
➤ Mouth ulcers
➤ Reducing sebum secretions in scalp

Dose:

The German Federal Institute of Pharmaceutical and Medicinal Products has established safety guidelines for the prolonged and unsupervised use of Licorice that should be adhered to. Take not more than the equivalent of 100 mg of glycyrrhizic acid daily (about 2-5 gm whole root).

For short term (four to six weeks), higher dose consumption, the German authorities consider up to 600 mg glycyrrhizin (5-15 gm whole root) safe for unsupervised consumption.

DGL tablets are to be chewed. Follow the manufacturer's package directions.

Cautions:

Glycyrrhizin may increase blood sodium and decrease potassium levels. Edema and slight rises in blood pressure may result. These effects are generally only seen with excessive doses (one study sighted 30-40 gm over 9 months), and may perhaps only be significant in the elderly or those suffering from renal, hepatic, or cardiovascular disease. While side effects are generally rare within normal doses, if swelling of the face or ankles occurs, or if muscle weakness is experienced, the dose should be lowered or consumption stopped. If necessary, you may consider supplementing with extra potassium to offset this effect.

If one has high blood pressure or a propensity to high blood pressure, cardiovascular disease, abnormalities of heart rhythm, kidney disease, or is taking medication that may lower potassium levels, use Licorice with caution. The DGL form is often used to avoid this problem if using Licorice for ulcers.

It should also be noted that adverse effects are more likely to occur when clinical tests are conducted with isolated glycyrrhizin or a semi-synthetic analog of it. When glycyrrhizin is ingested as part of a Licorice extract, its bioavailability is decreased due to some interaction between it and other Licorice components during the intestinal absorption process. Taking an extract is clearly safer than isolating a drug-like component of the plant.

Another fear that has cropped up recently is that of men reducing their testosterone levels by taking Licorice. In an Italian study, men ages 22-24 years of age were given 7 gm of Licorice per day containing 500 mg of Glycyrrhizic Acid. Their testosterone levels dropped. However, look to see where this is on the scale of responsible Licorice ingestion. Remember the rule. Less than 100 mg of glycyrrhizic acid per day. At these levels, the risk of decreased libido or sexual dysfunction is unlikely.

References:

See General Resources

Abe, N, et al. "Interferon Induction by Glycyrrhizin and Glycyrrhetinic Acid in Mice." *Microb Immunol*. 1982; 26:535-539

Acharya, S, et al. "A Preliminary Open Trial on Interferon Stimulator Derived From Glycyrrhiza Glabra in the Treatment o Subacute Hepatic Failure." *Indian J Med Res*. 1993; 98:69-74

Arase, U, et al. "The Long-Term Efficacy of Glycyrrhizin in Chronic Hepatitis C Patients." *Cancer*. 1997; 79:1494-1500

Armanini, D, et al. "Reduction of Serum Testosterone in Men by Licorice." *New Engl J Med*. 1999; 341:1158

Baschetti, R. "Chronic Fatigue Syndrome and Licorice." *New Zealand Medical Journal*. 1995; 156-7

Cantelli-Forti, G, et al. "Interaction of Licorice on Glycyrrhizin Pharmacokinetics." *Environmental Health Perspectives*. 1994; 120:65-68

Chang, H, ed. *Pharmacology and Applications of Chinese Materia Medica*. Philadelphia. World Scientific. 1986

Chandler, R. "Licorice, More Than Just a Flavor." *Can Pharm J*. 1985; 118:421-4

Csonka, G, et al. "Treatment of Herpes Genitals with Carbonoxolone and Cicloxolone Creams-A Double Blind Placebo Controlled Study." *Br J Ven Dis*. 1984; 60:178-81

Cyong, J. "A Pharmacological Study of the Anti-Inflammatory Activity of Chinese Herbs. A Review." *Acupunct Electro Ther*. 1982; 7:173-202

Davis, E, et al. "Medicinal Uses of Licorice through the Millennia: the Good and Plenty of It." *Mol Cell Endocrinol*. 1991; 78:1-6

DerMarderosian, A, ed. *Review of Natural Products*. St. Louis, MO, Facts and Comparisons, 1999

Evans, F. "The Rational Use of Glycyrrhetinic Acid in Dermatology." *Br J Clin Pract*. 1958; 12:269-279

Farese, R, et al. "Licorice Induced Hypermineralocorticoidism." *N Engl J Med*. 1991; 325:1223-1227

Foster, S, Tyler, V. *Tylers Honest Herbal: A Sensible Guide to the Use of Herbs and Related Remedies*. Rochester, VT. Healing Arts Press. 1999

Gibson, M. "Glycyrrhiza in Old and New Perspectives." *Lloydia*. 1978; 41:348-354

Hattori, T, et al. "Preliminary Evidence for Inhibitory Effect of Glycyrrhizin on HIV Replication in Patients With AIDS." *Antiviral Res*. 1989; 11:255-262

Ikegami, N, et al. "Prophylactic Effect of Long Term Oral Administration of Glycyrrhizin on AIDS Development of Asymptomatic Patients." *Int Conf AIDS*. 1993; 9:234

Kumagai, A, et al. "Effect of Glycyrrhizin on Estrogen Action." *Endocrinol J*. 1967; 14:34-38

Kumagai, A, et al. "Effects of Glycyrrhizin on Thymolytic and Immunosuppressive

Action of Cortisone." *Endocrinol J*. 1967; 14:39-42

Kuroyanagi, T, et al. "Effect of Prednisolone and Glycyrrhizin on Passive Transfer of Experimental Allergic Encephalomyelitis." *Allergy*. 1966; 15:67-75

Matsumoto, T, et al. "Effect of Licorice Roots on Carrageenan-Induced Decrease in Immune Complexes Clearance in Mice." *Journal of Ethnopharmacology*. 1996; 53:1-4

Morgan, A, et al. "Comparison Between Cimetidine and Caved-S® in the Treatment of Gastric Ulceration, and Subsequent Maintenance Therapy." *Gut*. 1982; 23:545-51

Mori, K, et al. "Effects of Glycyrrhizin in Hemophilia Patients with HIV-1 Infection. *Tohoku J Exp Med*. 1990; 162:183-93

Poswillo, D, et al. "Management of Recurrent Aphthous Ulcers." *Br Dent J*. 1984; 157:55-57

Reed, P, et al. "Comparative Study on Carbonoxolone and Cimetidine in the Management of Duodenal Ulcer." *Acta Gastro Enerol Belgica*. 1983; 46:459-468

Rees, W, et al. "Effect of DGL on Gastric Mucosal Damage by Aspirin." *Scand J Gastroenterol*. 1979; 14:605-607

Sigurjonsdottir, H, et al. *J Human Hyperten*. 1995; 9:345-48 Name of article missing Will check out

Stormer, F, et al. "Glycyrrhizic Acid in Licorice-Evaluation of Health Hazard." *Fd Chem Toxicol*. 1993; 31:303-312

Maca

(Lepidium meyenii)

Other Common Names:

Maka, Maca-Maca, Peruvian Ginseng

Background:

Maca is a perennial plant of the Andean mountains. It grows between an elevation of 11,000 and 14,500 feet. The Inca Indians domesticated it about 2,000 years ago. To them, it was a very valuable commodity. Because so little can grow in the inhospitable regions in which they lived, they used Maca to trade for staples like rice, corn and beans, with tribes that lived at lower elevations.

Native Peruvians have utilized Maca roots both as a food and as a medicine. As a food, it probably has more nutritional value than any other food crop grown there. It is rich in sugars, protein, starches, and essential minerals. It can be eaten fresh or dried. Fresh, it is baked or roasted much like a potato. Dried, it can be stored for up to seven years. After that, you can slice it thin and pave walkways with it (just kidding). Before the seven years are up, the dried root is boiled in milk or water to make porridge. Mountain people are big on porridge. I can remember mountain climbing in Africa; my Chaga guide fed me their special porridge called *Ugali*, after which I developed a distinct liking for wallpaper paste. In addition to porridge, or wallpaper paste, they often make a popular sweet fermented drink called *Maca Chicha*, which I may try when I go climbing in the Andes.

Medicinally, Maca has been used for enhancing overall vigor and fertility for centuries. When the Spanish conquered South America, they found that the farm animals they brought with them from Spain were reproducing poorly in the highlands. The local Indians recommended feeding the animals Maca root, which proved to be successful in enhancing their fertility. The Indians probably should have kept their mouths shut, and history might have turned out differently.

In addition to reproductive and sexual disorders, in Peruvian herbal medicine, Maca is also used for menstrual disorders, menopause symptoms, as an immunostimulant, for anemia, tuberculosis, stomach cancer, mental clarity, increased energy, stamina and endurance, as well as to enhance memory.

Science:

Maca's fertility enhancing properties were actually validated in rats in the 60s, when researchers discovered it increased fertility in laboratory test animals. However, the real breakthrough research in this area was published in a major peer-reviewed medical journal, *Urology*, in April of 2000.

In this study, mice fed a specific extract of Maca, standardized to two of its actives, macamides & macaenes, exhibited a significant increase in sexual activity when compared to a control group. Additional toxicity testing revealed no untoward pharmacological effects, just very tired mice. Researchers concluded that Maca promotes libido, sexual potency and energy, and that it may be useful in the treatment of age-related sexual dysfunction. Anecdotal reports from individuals using this extract seem to further confirm an increase in libido, enhanced sexual function, and increased frequency of sex.

Since the Inca's fed Maca to their warriors to impart "kallpa" or strength, it has been sought after to increase energy, stamina and endurance. This is probably why it is referred to as Peruvian ginseng. Chacon, who wrote a book that is considered the definitive study on Maca, isolated alkaloids that he believes work on the hypothalamus-pituitary axis, modulating (up-regulating) adrenal activity. Remember the adrenals are the glands that manufacture your flight, fright, fight hormones.

Modern Day Uses:

Modern day uses are probably no different than Maca's ancient uses. They include:

> ➢ Aphrodisiac
> ➢ Fertility

> ➢ Impotence
> ➢ Erectile dysfunction
> ➢ Vitality
> ➢ Menopause & Menstruation
> ➢ Mental clarity
> ➢ Chronic Fatigue Syndrome
> ➢ General immunity
> ➢ Anabolic steroid alternative

Dose:

Since Maca has traditionally been used as a food, supplemental doses have previously been almost impractical. Five to twenty grams twice daily would not have been unusual. That would mean taking five to twenty one-gram capsules twice daily. However, with the introduction of concentrated extracts standardized to .6% macamides & macaenes, the same benefits may be attained with 500 mg twice daily.

Cautions:

None known

References:

See General Resources

Chacon, G. "La Importancia de Maca en la Alimentacion y Salud del ser Jumano y Animal 2,000 Anos Antes y Despues de Cristo y en el Siglo XXI. Peru, 1997

Chacon, G. "La Maca y su Habitat." *Revista Peruana de Biologia.* 1990; 3:171-2

Dini, A, et al. "Chemical Composition of Lepidium meyenii." *Food Chemistry.* 1994; 49:347-49

Johns, T. "The Anu and the Maca." *Journal of Ethnobiology.* 1981; 1:208-212

King, S. "Ancient Buried Treasure of the Andes." *Garden.* 1986; Nov/Dec

Leon, J. "The Maca (Lepidium Meyenii) a Little Known Food Plant of Peru." *Economic Botany.* 1964; 18:122-27

Quiros, C, et al. "Physiological Studies and Determination of Chromosome Number in Maca, Lepidium meyenii." *Economic Botany*. 1996; 50:216-23

Walker, M. "Medical Journalist's Report of Innovative Biologics: Effects of Peruvian Maca on Hormonal Functions." 1998; *Townsend Letter for Doctors & Patients*. Nov

Milk Thistle

(Silybum marianum)

Other Common Names:

Carduus marianus, Mary Thistle, Marian Thistle, Lady's Thistle, Our Lady's Thistle, Holy Thistle, Wild Artichoke

Background:

Milk Thistle is a plant indigenous to Kashmir and the Mediterranean, grows wild throughout Europe, and behaved itself, studied hard, got a Green Card, and became naturalized in California, the eastern United States, and Australia.

As a food, Milk Thistle was once grown for its leaves in salads, its flowers to be eaten as artichokes are, and for its seeds as a coffee substitute. Medicinally, it has been use for over 2,000 years.

The common name, milk thistle, is derived from the milky white veins on the leaves, which, when broken open, yield a milky sap. The genus name, Silybum, is derived from the name given to edible thistles by Dioscorides, the Greek physician of the 1st century AD. And, the species name, marianum, comes from the legend that the white mottling on the leaves came from a drop of the Virgin Mary's milk. And, perhaps the most widespread folk use of this plant has been in assisting the nursing mother in the production of milk. This also explains Milk Thistle's common names that refer to Mary and Holy.

There is confusion as to which part of the plant is used to formulate Milk Thistle medicinal preparations. Most literature published in English refers to the seed as the plant part used, even thought it is the fruit which has the greatest concentration of valuable phytochemicals. Well, the seeds, that are being referred to, are the fruit; they just look like seeds. They are small hard fruits technically know as achenes (small, dry, one-seeded fruits with a thin wall that don't split open at maturity) from which a feathery cluster has been removed.

Milk Thistle's use as a liver drug goes back to the Greeks and Pliny the Elder (23-79 AD), who wrote that it was excellent for "carrying off bile." Culpepper (1616-1654), England's superstar herbalist, found Milk Thistle useful for decongesting the liver and spleen, and good against jaundice. In the U.S. at the turn of the 20th century, the Eclectics, in addition to treating liver obstructions with Milk Thistle, used it for varicose veins, menstrual problems, and disorders for the spleen and kidneys.

As most herbal drugs fell from favor in the early 20th century, so did Milk Thistle. However, leave it to the Europeans to get us back on track. In the 1960s, heavy research on Milk Thistle's liver protecting properties was being conducted in Germany. In 1968, Wagner, Horhammer, and Munster identified and isolated the active bioflavonoid complex, calling it *silymarin*. Silymarin is what gives Milk Thistle it's medicinal benefits, and appropriately, the term has become interchangeable with "Milk Thistle extract."

Science:

Silymarin is one of the most potent liver protecting substances known to man, and as a result thereof, has become the focus of hundreds of clinical studies. It is primarily a mixture of the substances collectively called flavonlignans; and the primary constituents are silybin (silibinin), silychristin (silichristin), and silidianin (silidyanin), the most biologically active being silybin. I think they should do a few studies on how to best spell these substances.

Silymarin has hepatoprotective, antihepatotoxic, and antioxidant properties. It passes freely from plasma to bile and concentrates in liver cells. Its mechanisms of action are best summarized as follows:

> ➢ It increases protein synthesis in liver cells by increasing the activity of nucleic acids. This results in the activation of the regenerative capacity of the liver.

> ➢ It alters the outer layer of liver cells, so as to disallow the entrance of toxins. It does this by blocking the binding sites, thus inhibiting the uptake.

➢ It has antioxidant properties, scavenges for free radicals and increases the intracellular concentration of glutathione, an endogenous antioxidant essential to many Phase II liver detoxification reactions.

➢ It may also inhibit the carcinogenic effects of PGE2 prostaglandins.

As a hepatoprotectant, Silymarin has been shown to block the toxic effects of poisonous mushrooms and hepatotoxic drugs like tetracycline, erythromycin, amitriptyine, nortriptyline, haloperidol, phenothiazine, butyrophenone, and acetaminophen.

Silymarin offers benefits to those with cirrhosis and hepatitis, ameliorating disease indices like elevated liver enzymes and bilirubin levels. Clinical trials consistently show histological improvements. Silymarin also has a hypolipidemic effect, decreasing total cholesterol by decreasing its synthesis in the liver.

Modern Day Uses:

Indications for Milk thistle are for any liver-based health problem. Because of its indisputable protective, regenerative, and antitoxic activity, Milk Thistle can be used for the following:

➢ Regenerate liver cells damaged by alcohol or drugs. It will only affect healthy cells, having no stimulating effect on cancer cells.

➢ Act as an adjunct to periodic body detoxification programs.

➢ Impede the advancement of cirrhosis.

➢ Complement the treatment of hepatitis.

➢ Protect against occupational liver poisons.

➢ Protect the liver against hepatotoxic pharmaceuticals, including the chemotherapy drug cisplatin.

Through other mechanisms, Milk Thistle may also be effective in treating psoriasis and gallstones. Psoriasis, among other things, is associated with excessive production of leukotrienes (mediators of inflammation), and an imbalance between the nucleotides cAMP, and cGMP. Silymarin reduces leukotriene formation, and down-regulates cGMP, bringing it back in balance with cAMP. It benefits gallstone production by increasing the solubility of bile.

Dose:

The concentration of Silymarin in crude Milk Thistle is only 1.5%-3%, and it is not very soluble in water. Additionally, research has demonstrated that low concentrations of silymarin are poorly absorbed. For these reasons, it is paramount to choose a highly concentrated and standardized extract to achieve the effects documented in the exhaustive list of clinical studies.

Standardized extracts of Milk Thistle are available in silymarin concentrations of 70-80%. However, you may still have to do some math to get a proper dose. The average dosage range is 280 to 420 mg daily, in divided doses, calculated as silymarin. One of the most common clinical doses is 420 mg of silymarin daily divided into three doses, and sustained for six to eight weeks. A maintenance dose might be considered 280 mg daily, divided into two doses.

For example, a daily dose of 600 mg of a Milk Thistle extract, standardized to 70% silymarin, yields 420 mg of actives. Or, a 175 mg capsule standardized to 80%, yields 140 mg of actives. Therefore, take one capsule three times daily, and you have your 420 mg.

Cautions:

There are no known interactions with other drugs. The only side effect that has been observed is a mild laxative effect with high doses, and this is only a transient effect, abating after a few days.

Diabetic patients taking Milk Thistle should carefully monitor their blood glucose. They may require less medication to avoid hypoglycemia.

Remember that liver disorders are not self-diagnosable diseases. Work with your doctor.

References:
See General Resources

Albrecht, M. et al. "Therapy of Toxic Liver Pathologies with Legalon®." *Z Klin Med.* 1992; 47:87-92

Awang, D. "Milk Thistle." *Can Pharm J.* 1993; 422:403-04

DiMario F. and Farini, L. et al. "The Effects of Silymarin on the Liver Function Parameters of Patients with Alcohol Induced Liver Disease: A Double Blind Study." *Der Toxish-Metabolische Herberschaden.* 1981; 54-58

Ferenci, P, et al. "Randomized Controlled Trial of Silymarin Treatment in Patients with Cirrhosis of the Liver." *J Hepatol.* 1989; 9:105-13

Flora, K. et al. "Milk Thistle For the Therapy of Liver Disease." *Am J Gastroenterol.* 1998; 93:139-43

Grungreiff, K, et al. "The Value of Drug Therapy For Liver Disease in General Practice." *Med Welt.* 1995; 46:222-7

Grieve, M. *A Modern Herbal.* New York, NY. Dover Publications. 1971

Hofer, J. *Wiener Klinische Wochenschrift.* 1983; 95:240-3

Lirussi, R, et al. "Cytoprotection in the Nineties: Experience with Ursodeoxycholic Acid and Silymarin in Chronic Liver Disease." *Acta Physiol Hungar.* 1992; 80:363-7

Monograph. *Alternative Medicine Review.* 1999; 4:272-274

Muriel, P. et al. "Silymarin Protects against Paracetamol Induced Lipid Peroxidation and Liver Damage." *J Appl Toxicol.* 1992; 12:439-442

Nassauto, G. et al. "Effect of Silibinin on Biliary Lipid Composition. Experimental and Clinical Study." *J Hepatol* 1991; 12:290-295

O'Hara, M, et al. "A Review of 12 Commonly Used Medicinal Herbs." *Arch Fam Med.* 1998; 7:523-536

Palasciano, G. et al. "The Effect of Silymarin on Plasma Levels of Malon-Dialdehyde in Patients Receiving Long-Term Treatment with Psychotropic Drugs." *Current Therapeutic Research* 1994; 55:537-45

Science News. 1985; 128:26-9

Salmi, H, et al. "Effect of Silymarin on Chemical, Functional and Morphological Alterations of the Liver." *Scand J Gastroent.* 1982; 17:517-21

Sonnenbichler, J. and Goldberg, M. et al. "Stimulating Effect of Silybin on the DNA Synthesis in Partially Hepatectomized Rat Livers: Non-response in Hepatoma and Other Malignant Cell Lines." *Biochem Pharmacol.* 1986; 35:538-541

Valenzuela, A, et al. "Selectivity of Silymarin on the Increase of the Glutathione Content in Different Tissues of the Rat." *Planta Med.* 1989 55:420-2

Wagner, H. et al. "The Chemistry of Silymarin (Silybin), the Active Principle of the Fruits of Silybum marianum." *Arzneim-Forsch Drug Res.* 1968; 18:688-96

Nettles

(Urtica dioica)

Other Common Names:
Stinging Nettle, Common Nettle, Greater Nettle, Ortie, Urtica

Background:
Nettles grow wild in temperate regions of the world. The genus name Urtica comes from the Latin meaning, "to burn." As one of the many who have brushed up against this plant on a hike, I can relate! They say that the antidote for the sting is in the plant. However, what they, whoever they are, don't say is how you get it out without touching the plant again.

They also say that rubbing fresh Dock, which often grows in the neighborhood, will reduce the stinging. There is an old rhyme that goes: *Nettle in, dock out. Dock rub, nettle out!* The sting may also be reduced by rubbing Rosemary, Mint or Sage on the affected area. I say, give it up. Suck it in and move on. Life is too short.

The flowers of Nettles are curious. They are incomplete. The male flowers have only stamens (pollen producing organs). The female flowers have only pistils (seed producing organs). These male and female flowers usually are found on only one plant, either a female plant, or a male plant. This is how Nettle got its species name, *dioica*, which means "two houses."

In the second and third centuries BC, Nettles were used as an antidote for poisons, snakebite, and insect stings. I don't know whether they beat it out of you, or if the treatment was internal. The Greek masters used nettles as a diuretic, laxative, asthma, pleurisy, and for ailments of the spleen. In addition, the Romans used it to stop bleeding. In England, Nettles are said to have been introduced by the Romans. When Julius Caesar landed in Britain, a climate considerably more harsh than home, his soldiers brought Nettles with which to flog themselves. This was their means of staying warm. North American Natives used Nettle as an anti-rheumatic, and Eastern Indians still use it for uterine hemorrhaging, skin eruptions, and nosebleeds.

When Germany and Austria starting running short of cotton, during World War I, Nettles were considered for a substitute. Perhaps they knew that Nettle plants were used in the Bronze Age to make burial shrouds. In 1916, tests showed that there was strong potential for the widespread use of Nettle cloth. It proved as good or better than cotton for many uses. A couple pair of German overalls recovered in 1917 showed them to be made of Cotton and two species of Nettle. What a novel idea to have your clothes also be your heater.

Extracts of the leaves have been used topically for the treatment of rheumatic disorders, hair loss, eczema, as an astringent, styptic, and wound healer. And, Nettle is high in iron, although I can't imagine consuming vast quantities of plant material when such good iron supplements are available today (look for HemIron).

Science:

The primary chemical component of Nettles leaf is agglutinin, however, the plant's silica level seems to be the compound of choice for the standardization of the extract. On the other hand, one of the up and coming uses of Nettles, benign prostatic hypertrophy, utilizes the root, and a specific lectin may be the ingredient to which these extracts are standardized. The "stinging" compounds in the leaf include formic acid, histamine, and serotonin, and these compounds may also be considered active. Nettles are very complicated.

Nettles' gout treating benefits are believed to come from its ability to mobilize and excrete uric acid through the kidneys.

Nettles contain several anti-inflammatory compounds, such as cyclooxygenase and lipooxygenase inhibitors, and substances that affect the secretion of cytokines. Cytokines are substances released by cells under attack, as messengers to alert adjoining cells to prepare for attack by releasing a host of troublesome chemicals. The result is an immune response that contributes to inflammation. Human studies have confirmed that concomitant use of Nettles and nonsteroidal anti-inflammatory drugs results in a dramatic reduction of the amount of drug necessary to treat arthritis.

One human study has been done in Oregon on "freeze dried" Nettles, suspiciously close to where there is a manufacturer of "freeze dried" Nettles. In this 69-person study, 57 percent of the subjects rated Nettles moderately to highly effective for allergy symptoms. Thirty-seven percent of the placebo group rated "nothing" (placebo) moderately to highly effective. Forty-three percent of the Nettles group found the extract ineffective. These are not overwhelming results, and I know of no more studies completed. However, I understand how frustrated allergy sufferers are, and would say it's worth a try to give Nettles a go.

The root extract, as mentioned above, is getting a lot of attention for the treatment of benign prostatic hypertrophy. The mechanism by which it may exert its action is by inhibiting the potassium ATP-ase activity of the prostate. The net result of this mechanism is that prostatic cell proliferation is suppressed. Human studies show Nettle Root increases urinary flow rates and decreases residual urine volumes. Nettle Root works by a different mechanism from which other botanicals work on the prostate, making it a great secondary or tertiary ingredient in a prostate combination formula.

Modern Day Uses:
The best known uses of Nettles are for the treatment of:

> Gout
> Arthritic and rheumatic conditions
> To reduce the amount of nonsteroidal anti-inflammatory drugs needed for arthritis
> Diuretic
> Urinary stones
> Perhaps allergies
> Benign prostatic hypertrophy (root extract)

German health authorities have approved Nettles for the use of:

> Irrigation therapy for diseases of the lower urinary tract

> ➢ Diuretic
> ➢ Prevention of kidney gravel
> ➢ Supportive therapy for rheumatic ailments

Dose:
Use the manufacturer's label recommendations.

Cautions:
The German Federal Institute of Pharmaceutical and Medicinal Products lists no known side effects or contraindications. Common sense would dictate not using Nettles with other diuretic drugs.

References:
See General Resources

Chrubasik, S, et al. Evidence for Anti-rheumatic Effectiveness of Herba Rricae Dioicae in Acute Arthritis: A Pilot Study. *Phytomedicine*. 1997; 4:105-108

Hartman, R, et al. "Inhibition of 5 Alpha Reductase and Aromatase by PHL-00801 (Prostatonin®), a Combination of PY 102 (Pygeum Africanum) and UklR 102 (Urtica Dioica) Extracts." *Phytomedicine*. 1996; 2:121-128

Konrad, L, et al. "Antiproliferative Effect on Human Prostate Cancer Cells by a Stinging Nettle Root Extract." *Planta Med*. 2000; 66:44-47

Mittman, P. "Randomized, Double-Blind Study of Freeze Dried Urtica Dioico I the Treatment of Allergic Rhinitis." *Planta Medica*. 1990; 56:44-7

Urticae Herba, Urticae Follium, Urticae Radix. ESCOP Monograph, 1997

Wagner, H, et al. "Search for the Antiprostatic Principle of Stinging Nettle (Urtica Dioica) Roots. *Phytomedicine*. 1994; 1::213-224

Noni

(Morinda citrifolia)

Other Common Names:
Nonu, Nono, Indian Mulberry,

Background:
The benefits of Noni have been known in Chinese, Caribbean, and South Pacific history as far back as the Han dynasty 2,000 years ago. Since the ancestors of today's Polynesians most likely migrated to Hawaii from Southeast Asia, it stands to reason that these first settlers would bring with them plants and animals they would need to survive in a new land.

Many plants may have been brought for food, but others must certainly have been brought for medicines. This is how it is believed that Noni found its way to Hawaii. A retrospective of traditional Hawaiian herbal medicine finds Noni one of the most mentioned remedies. Kahunas, traditional medicine men, have used the leaves, bark, flowers and fruit of Noni for literally hundreds of health maladies. It is actually considered a sacred plant.

There are many old Polynesian tales about Noni. One is a tale of Kamapua'a, the pig god, who loved Pele, the volcano goddess. The pig god taunted Pele with the chant, "I have seen the woman gathering Noni-Scratching Noni-Pounding Noni." The chant was supposed to have referred to Pele's eyes, which were red. She became so angry that she plunged into battle with him. Not exactly the material that movies are made out of, but nonetheless a tale. And, what is a pig god? A Tongan myth recounts that the god Maui was restored to life by having the leaves of Noni placed on his body. Definitely a more elegant yarn than the pig god story.

Science:
What makes Noni tick has remained elusive. The most interesting information available comes from Dr. Ralph M. Heinicke at the Uni-

versity of Hawaii in, to the best of my knowledge, unpublished research. Dr. Heinicke believes that Noni's actives have not been identified because they are not present in the plant. They are formed after the fruit has been ingested.

In previous research on bromelain, Dr. Heinicke identified a new alkaloid that he named "xeronine." Using the same techniques, he was able to isolate the same compound from Noni. According to Heinicke, xeronine is a small alkaloid active in the trillionth of a gram range. It occurs in all healthy animal and plant cells. Even though Noni fruit has negligible amounts of free xeronine, Dr. Heinicke claims it has appreciable amounts of its precursor, which he has named "proxeronine."

By his own admission, Dr. Heinicke recognizes that many years of research are going to be required to demonstrate how xeronine functions in the body and how Noni fits into the picture, but in the meantime, he is putting forth a possible hypothesis.

Dr. Heinicke believes that in addition to xeronine and proxeronine, Noni also contains the inactive form of the enzyme that converts proxeronine to xeronine. Observations that Noni not taken on an empty stomach yields few pharmacological reactions lead him to postulate that taking it on an empty stomach activates this enzyme.

Dr. Heinicke proposes that the primary function of xeronine is to regulate the rigidity and shape of specific proteins. Since these proteins have different functions, it explains why a single substance can have such a wide range of often unrelated responses on the body. This thinking would also explain the diverse actions of many botanical medicines, like Ginseng, if not all, herbal medicines.

The action which xeronine has on the body would depend on which tissues might be low in it, and theoretically, any disease or subset of disease could be alleviated by bringing xeronine levels up. However, Dr. Heinicke is clear that xeronine will not be a panacea for any and all diseases. Only if the disease is specifically caused by a lack of xeronine will supplemental xeronine alleviate the symptoms of the problem.

Heinicke proposes that each tissue has cells, which have proteins, which in turn have receptor sites for the absorption of xeronine. A number of these proteins are inert forms of enzymes that require absorbed xeronine to become active. Now, if you accept this hypotheses, then you can further theorize that xeronine converts procollagenase into specific protease, which removes dead tissue from burns. And, now you have the mechanism by which Noni, or Aloe for that matter, is an effective treatment for burns.

Other proteins might be activators of endorphins, which would explain Noni's "feel good" or pain relieving effects. Or, if the proteins that formed the pores in the intestines or blood vessels were re-shaped, perhaps Noni's effect on digestion could be explained.

It should be noted that Heinecke's findings have been exploited heavily by multi level marketers, and he has lent his approval to one commercial product. However, some biochemists familiar with the research have dismissed it almost immediately as methodologically flawed. Heinecke's findings have not been confirmed by other researchers, who continue to regard "xeronine" as suspect. At the very best, we can only regard his work as theoretical.

Nonetheless, modern science is just now starting to look at Noni. From studies done in the 1990s, one can draw the following conclusions:

> ➤ Noni may retard tumor growth by stimulating the immune system.
> ➤ Noni constituents may work at the cellular level to regenerate and enhance cell function.
> ➤ Noni has been shown to relieve pain.
> ➤ Noni had a significant impact on arresting implanted pre-cancerous cells.
> ➤ Noni has antiseptic activity.
> ➤ Noni is antibacterial, antifungal, and antiparasitic.

Modern Day Uses:
An interesting game might be to try and guess something that Noni is

not good for. A list of purported benefits for which there is some scientific documentation is as follows: This does not include the countless folklore uses.

> ➤ Pain (often called the pain killer tree)
> ➤ Headache including migraine (often called the headache tree)
> ➤ Infections (various including cold, flu, sinus, sore throat, cough, fever, mouth and gum)
> ➤ Diarrhea
> ➤ Intestinal worms
> ➤ Arthritis
> ➤ Backache
> ➤ Wound healing
> ➤ Cancer prevention
> ➤ High blood pressure
> ➤ Diabetes (adult onset)
> ➤ Immune enhancement

If you were to add in the additional disorders that Dr. Heinicke believes might be helped by Noni, the list would also include menstrual cramps, sprains, mental depression, senility, poor digestion, gastric ulcers, atherosclerosis, and addiction.

Dose:

Since real Noni juice smells and tastes terrible, so disagreeable most people would never take a second dose, I suggest the use of a freeze-dried tablet or capsule. Juices on the market today must be pasteurized. The heat involved tends to dis-configure the protein chains that impart Noni's health benefits, decreasing its effectiveness. Not to mention the doctoring required to hide the taste.

Additionally, if pepsin and stomach acid destroy the enzymes that liberate xeronine, as Dr. Heinicke suggests, it would make sense to take it on an empty stomach with water to discourage a lengthy stay.

Follow the manufacturer's label recommendations.

Cautions:
None known.

References:
See General Resources

Dixon A, McMillen H, Etkin N, *Economic Botany* (1999) 53(1):51-68.

Hirazumi, A. et al. "Anticancer Activity of Morinda citrifolia on Intraperitoneally Implanted Lewis Lung Carcinoma in Syngenic Mice." *Porc West Pharmacol Soc.* 1994; 37:145-146

Hiramatsu, T. et al. "Induction of Normal Phenotypes in RAS-Transformed Cells by Damnacanthal From Morinda citrifolia." *Cancer Letters.* 1993; 73:161-66

Schechter, S. "Nonu: Nature's True Adaptogen From The South Pacific." *Total Health.* 1999; 21:40-41

Younoa, C. et al. "Analgesic and Behavioral Effects of Morinda citrifolia." *Planta Medica.* 1990; 56:430-434

Oats

(Avena sativa)

Other Common Names:
Groats, Haver, Haver-Corn, Haws

Background:
After having probably originating in Northeast Africa, the Mediterranean and China, and having been cultivated back to 2000 BC, Oats today is primarily grown in the United States, Canada, Russia and Germany. It derived from wild grasses and has evolved into what it is today.

The remains of the plant have been found in the digestive tracts of prehistoric man, so at the very least, Oats must have played a role as a food source. Dioscorides, the 1st century AD Greek physician, wrote about Oats and its usefulness as a "cataplasm" (poultice) to treat coughs.

Traditionally, Oats have been used as a nutritive, demulcent remedy for chronic constipation, as an antispasmodic, and in baths for arthritis and inflammatory skin problems. However, outside its most widespread use today as a food to lower cholesterol, Oats claim to fame has been in the area of nervous disorders, namely nervous exhaustion and other nervous disabilities.

Perhaps Oats' use as a restorative from nervous prostration led to the expression "feeling one's oats." Or, could the cliché come from the fact that in China, Oats are used to regenerate the male reproductive system. There is even some interest in the use of Oats to stimulate female libido.

Science:
Oats contain polyphenols, saponins, gluten, mono- and oligosaccharides, various minerals, flavones, beta-glucans, and soluble and insoluble dietary fibers. Different components of Oats come into play

for each of its three primary categorical uses.

As a food, Oats have become a sound way of controlling and lowering blood fats. Oats fiber content binds cholesterol and bile salts in the intestine, blocking cholesterol absorption. These soluble fibers may also be fermented in the gut into a substance that is absorbed and then interferes with the synthesis of cholesterol.

Topically, Oats' gluten content has made it an effective aid in the management of itchy skin conditions. The market is peppered with over-the-counter remedies for the skin including colloidal oatmeal bath mixtures, soaps, and cosmetic products.

And then there is the work done with extracts of Oatstraw (the Oat remains left from the harvest) and extracts of Oat greens. These are generally where the medicinals are derived.

Fascinating research was born from the Chinese use of Oats for hormonal restoration. Modern science now has a clue to substantiate the use. Oats does have a potential influence on reproductive hormones based on its ability to stimulate the release of luteinizing hormone from a brain gland, at least in animal studies. Since luteinizing hormone stimulates the release of testosterone, and testosterone is the primary sex hormone for male performance and female libido, a link has been made.

Oats seems to reduce the number of cigarettes smoked per day and diminishes the craving for cigarettes. One study showed that over a 28-day period, habitual smokers were able to reduce the number of cigarettes they smoked from 19.5 per day to 5.7 per day. This was while the cigarette consumption in the placebo group remained constant. This effect carried for two months beyond the scope to the study.

Another study on addiction, this time morphine, was based on an Indian traditional remedy for addiction. In this study, an Oat extract was administered to ten chronic users. At the end of the treatment, which averaged 34 days, six gave up morphine completely, two reduced their intake, and two remained hooked. No serious withdrawal symptoms or side effects were noted.

Modern Day Uses:

Consider Oat extracts as:

- ➢ Nervous system restorative
- ➢ Convalescence
- ➢ Strengthen a weakened constitution
- ➢ Anxiety
- ➢ Stress
- ➢ Nerve disorders
  - o Shingles
  - o Herpes
  - o Multiple Sclerosis
  - ➢ Male sexual restorative
  - ➢ Female libido
  - ➢ Tobacco and drug addiction and withdrawal

Consider Oat topically for:

- ➢ Dry skin
- ➢ Eczema
- ➢ Inflammatory skin conditions
- ➢ Itching skin

Use Oat Bran as a food for:

- ➢ Lowering cholesterol
- ➢ Preventing gallstones
- ➢ Reducing colon cancer risk
- ➢ Irritable bowel syndrome
- ➢ Diverticulosis
- ➢ Chronic constipation

Dose:

Oat Bran: Most studies use 50 to 100 g of dietary fiber daily.
Topically: Use once or twice daily.
Extract: Follow manufacturer's directions.

Cautions:

If you are not used to dietary fiber, expect to have a little transitory bloating, fullness, flatulence, and increased bowel movements.

References:

See General Resources

Anand, C. "Effect of Avena Sativa on Cigarette Smoking." *Nature*. 1971; 233:496

Anand, C. "Treatment of Opium Addiction." *Brit Med J*. 1971; 3:640

Connor, J, et al. "The Pharmacology of Avena Sativa." *J Pharm Pharmacol*. 1975; 27:92-98

DerMarderosian, A ed. *Review of Natural Products*. St. Louis, MO, Facts and Comparisons, 1999

Fukushima, M, et al. "Extraction and Purification of a Substance with Luteinizing Hormone Releasing Activity for the Leave of Avena Satva." *Tohuku J Exp Med*. 1976; 119:115-122.

Schmidt, K, et al. "Pharmcotherapy with Avena Sativa – A Double Blind Study." *Int J Clin Pharmacol*. 1976; 14:214-216

Olive Leaf

(Olea europaea)

Other Common Names:
Tree of Life, Olivier

Background:
The cultivation of olive trees goes back to about 3500 BC in Crete. The antiseptic benefits of the leaves must have been realized because the Cretans used them to clean wounds. Olive leaves have long been a symbol of peace, goodness and purity. My first thought of olive leaves is that of a peace symbol worn by ancient Greeks, but my most vivid memory is that of a girl I dated in the 60s who also wore them, and me with my love beads. The olive tree even worked its way into the Bible. Moses exempted from military service, young men who worked at the cultivation of the trees. Could this have been the first form of draft dodging?

In the 1800s, a tea made of olive leaves was used to treat stubborn fevers and malaria, and in the 1900s, a component of the leaf was found to help people resist disease.

The Latin name "olea" comes from the Greek word for olive, and "europaeus" refers to the chief area where this species was found, i.e., Europe. Olive trees are native to the Mediterranean but can be grown anywhere with similar climate.

Science:
The primary active constituent olive leaf contains is called oleuropein, and if you purchase this herb, you want to see the product standardized to this ingredient. Interestingly enough, this is the bitter element that is removed from olives when they are processed. It is also believed that this compound is what helps protect the tree from disease and insect attack.

Blood pressure, blood sugar, anti-microbial

Three areas on which research has focused include blood pressure, blood sugar, and anti-microbial effects. In animal studies, oleuropein has consistently shown an anti-hypertensive effect. It increases coronary output and is a vasodilator, probably via its effect on smooth muscle. It has also demonstrated antiarrhythmic properties. This is fine and dandy if you are a rabbit, cat, or a dog, but, for some reason, not so much if you're a rat. The conservative view here is that these effects are probably insignificant in humans, although the use of olives comes up in Italian folk medicine for such indications. I would not recommend throwing out your blood pressure medicine just yet, but for very mild cases of hypertension which should better be treated with diet and exercise, olive leaf may provide some beneficial effects. Because of oleuropeins' antioxidant activity, it has been shown to interfere with the biochemistry implicated in atherogenetic heart disease, as does vitamin E. This is a good thing.

Again in animal studies, olive leaf potentiates glucose-induced insulin release, in addition to enhancing the peripheral uptake of glucose. This results in a hypoglycemic effect. This could also be a good thing, but at this time, I don't think there is enough data to support the therapeutic use of olive leaf for diabetes.

The last significant area to look at is olive leaf's anti-microbial effects, and its possible use for chronic fatigue syndrome, colds, flu, herpes, AIDS-related problems, and more. I was amazed to learn that a giant drug company did much of the research validating the salt of oleuropein's (calcium elenolate) antiviral activity. They found it to be virucidal for all viruses against which it was tested. They believed that the protein coat of the virus was being compromised. Additionally, they felt it interfered with critical amino acid production, prevented virus spreading by inhibiting shedding, budding or assembly at the cell membrane, and directly interfered with the viruses' ability penetrate cells.

Later studies by others showed oleuropein effective at killing bacteria. They found it to damage bacterial cell membranes, causing intracellular matter to leak out. Other researchers tout olive leaf extract for its ability to support the immune system. That is, it can stimulate phago-cytosis, the ingestion and destruction of harmful foreign substances by immune cells called macrophages.

Modern Day Uses:
Possible uses of olive leaf extract are: viral infections (including Epstein-Barr), bacterial infections, yeast infections, parasites, and general immune support and well being.

Dose:
I recommend using a standardized extract containing not less than 10% oleuropein. Take 1000 mg three times daily for acute conditions. Take 500 mg once or twice daily as a preventative.

Cautions:
According to Commission E, there are no risks associated with the use of olive leaf. However, it is possible that some people may get some gastric irritation with larger doses. If this occurs, simply take it after meals. If you are using a product with a delivery system that bypasses the stomach, don't worry about it at all.

As a caution to diabetics, I would recommend watching your blood sugar a little more closely due to the possible hypoglycemic effect that may occur.

For those on medication for high blood pressure, monitor a little more closely while on Olive leaf extract.

References:
See General Resources

Visioli, F. et al. *Waste Waters from Olive Oil Production are Rich in Natural Antioxidants*. Basel: Virkauser Verlag, 1995

Juven, B. et al. Studies on the Mechanism of the Antimicrobial Action of Oleuropein. *J Appl Bact*. 1972

Tassou, C. et al. Effect of Phenolic Compounds and Oleuropein on the Germination of Bacillus Cereus T Spores. *Biotechnol Appl Biochem*. 1991. 13:231-237.

Tranter, H. et al. The Effect of the Olive Phenolic Compound, Oleuropein, on Growth and Enterotoxin B on Production by Staphylococcus Aureus. *J. Appl. Bact*. 1993. 74:253-259.

Elliott G. et al. Preliminary Studies with Calcium Elenalate, an Antiviral Agent. The Upjohn Co. Kalamazoo, Michigan. 1970.Elliott, G. et al. Preliminary Safety Studies with Calcium Elenolate, an Antiviral Agent. The Upjohn Co. Kalamazoo, Michigan. 1969

.Soret, M. Antiviral Activity of Calcium Elenolate on Parainfluenza Infections on Hamsters. Department of Virology Research. The Upjohn Co. Kalamazoo, Michigan. 1969.

Pygeum

(Prunus africana)

Other Common Names:
African Plum Tree

Background:
Pygeum is an evergreen native to the African forest. It can grow up to 150 in height. Interestingly, of the 200 species of the genus Prunus, only this tree is native to Africa. European interest goes back to the 1700s when medicine men from South African tribes shared its wonders for bladder pains with early settlers. They made a milk tea out of the bark and drank it to treat difficult urination. Colonists soon learned that African tribes people had been using the bark of this tree for hundreds of years for something called, "old man's disease."

Folkloric use led researchers to discover the use of Pygeum bark for the treatment of benign prostatic hyperplasia (BPH). In 1966, a Frenchman named Dr. Jacques Debat took out a patent on the extract, and in France, Pygeum has become the primary course for BHP. This is great for men with BPH, but it has not proven that great for the trees. It seems that bark collectors have become overzealous in their collection techniques and are leaving thousands of dead trees behind due to unsustainable harvesting. However, between close monitoring of the Convention on International Trade in Endangered Species (CITES), and the utilization of plantations, things are on guard.

Science:
Pygeum contains three groups of fat-soluble components, each with a different mechanism to combat BHP.

First, there are the phytosterols, exemplified by beta-sitosterol. The sterols have anti-inflammatory activity. Their mechanism of action is to interfere with the biosynthesis of inflammatory prostaglandins, namely PGE 2 and PGF 2-alpha.

Next there are the pentacyclic triterpenoids, exemplified by ursolic acid and oleanolic acid. The triterpenoids work by exerting a local diuretic effect. They inhibit the action of enzymes involved in the initial phase of inflammation. They strengthen the tiny veins and capillaries that would ordinarily leak and cause edema, allowing fluids to discharge instead.

The last group of actives is the linear acids, or ferulic esters, exemplified by n-docosanol and teracosanol. These guys reduce prolactin levels and block the accumulation of cholesterol in the prostate. This is important because prolactin increases the uptake of testosterone in the prostate, and cholesterol increases the binding sites for its troublesome metabolite dihydrotestosterone.

Pygeum may also increase prostate excretions. This may improve sexual function in those with compromised seminal fluid.

Modern Day Uses:
If you are a male, consider Pygeum for:

> ➤ Prostatitis
> ➤ Benign Prostate Hyperplasia
> ➤ Urine retention
> ➤ Frequent urination
> ➤ Difficult or painful urination
> ➤ Nocturnal urination
> ➤ Prostate cancer

Dose:
Research grade extracts are standardized to 13-15% triterpenes and have at least .5% n-docosanol. We used to recommend taking 100-200 mg daily in divided doses; however, recent medical studies have elucidated the effectiveness of a 100 mg, once daily dose.

Adjust your dose based on your positive outcome. Monitor your difficulty in urination, frequency of night time trips to the restroom, and your ability to completely empty your bladder. For those in need of extra help, consider using Pygeum with Saw Palmetto and/or Nettles.

Cautions:

Among the many clinical trials reported, Pygeum was found to have a low toxicity profile. There are some reports of gastrointestinal irritations manifested as stomach pain and nausea.

References:

See General Resources

Bassi, P, et al. "Standardized Extract of Pygeum Africanum in the Treatment of Benign Prostatic Hypertrophy." *Minerva Urologica.* 1987; 39:45

Breza, J, et al. "Efficacy and Acceptability of Pygeum Africanum Extract in the Treatment of Benign Prostatic Hyperplasia: A Multicenter Trial in Central Europe." *Curr Med Res Opin.* 1998; 14:127-139

Chatelain, C, et al. "Comparison of Once and Twice Daily Dosage Forms of Pygeum africanum Extract in Patients with Benign Prostatic Hyperplasia: A Randomized, Double-Blind Study, with Long-Term Open Label Extension." *Urology.* 1999; 54:473-8

Hartman, R, et al. "Inhibition of 5-alpha Reductase and Aromatase by a Combination of Pygeum Africanum and Urtica Dioica Extracts." *Phytomedicine.* 1996; 2:121-128

Krzeski, T, et al. "Combined Extracts of Urtica Dioica and Pygeum Africanum in the Treatment of Benign Prostatic Hyperplasia: Double-Blind Comparison of Two Doses." *Clin Ther.* 1993; 15:1011-20

Legramandi, C, et al. "Importance of Pygeum Africanum in the Treatment of Benign Prostatic Hypertrophy." *Gazz It Medical.* 1984; 143:73

Zurita, E, et al. "Treatment of Prostatic Hypertrophy with Extract Africana Prunus." *Rev Bras Med.* 1984; 41:48

Red Clover

(Trifolium pratense)

Other Common Names:

Purple Clover, Wild Clover, Meadow Clover, Honeysuckle Clover, Cleaver Grass, Marl Grass, Cow Grass, Beebread, Trefoil

Background:

The sweet smelling herb, Red Clover, while common to the United States and cultivated extensively in grasslands, is not native to us. It was brought here from Europe. At one time, the ancients burned it as incense to raise the spirits of the dead. The ancient Chinese dried the buds and stuffed them in pillows to enhance relaxation and invoke restful sleep. They also used a tea made with the fragrant blossoms as a deodorant before soap was commonplace. What could be more practical than a medicine that you can splash under your arms before you go to work?

The name Trifolium refers to the plant leaf, which generally comes in threes, but not always. Clover has a mystical following. Many people search for four leaf clovers and wear them for luck. In parts of Great Britain, leaves are worn as a charm to ward off evil and witches, and in Ireland, they have a thing called a shamrock.

Native Americans used Red Clover as a gargle for sore throats, whooping cough and asthma. But if you believe in the Doctrine of Signatures, the blossoms are red which suggests blood, and therefore a blood treatment. And, until the 1970s, Red Clover has been best known as a great "Alterative" herb.

Alteratives are a vague classification of herbs, much revered by herbalists and natural healers. They are substances that are believed to alter the blood and lymph system by their cleansing actions. Modern allopathic medicine rejects this concept, but it is still popular in the practices of alternative practitioners. The method by which Alteratives work is not generally agreed upon, but they are supposed to work on the liver and kidneys. Usually combined in formulae with other Alteratives like Burdock, Pau D'Arco, Licorice, Yellow Dock, and Black Cohosh, Alternative herbs are used to support everything from acne to cancer.

Science:
There is a new focus on Red Clover based on modern extraction techniques and the ability to concentrate potent active phytochemicals called isoflavones. Current research has shown that there are four isoflavones that play unique and important roles as phyto or phenolic estrogens. They are Genistein, Daidzein, Formononetin, and Biochanin.

Natural Estrogens
Phenolic estrogens are similar in structure to those made by the ovaries and are therefore able to mimic estrogenic activity. While they are a great deal weaker, they are actually able to benefit the body in both an estrogenic and anti-estrogenic manner, much like the drug raloxifene, a selective estrogen receptor modulator used to reduce the resorption of bone and treat osteoporosis. If levels of steroidal estrogen are high, isoflavones can displace them by competitive inhibition. That is, they can occupy estrogen receptor sites thus preventing the much stronger human estrogen from binding. If levels are low, like in menopause, these phytoestrogens can stand in and help allay the symptoms of deficiency.

Isoflavones, with over 1,000 different variants discovered so far, are largely restricted to the legume family, for example, chickpeas, lentils, beans and soy. This is why cultures that consume diets high in these foods enjoy health benefits we meat and dairy eating Westerners are just now discovering. Some of the most significant benefits isoflavones have to offer are antioxidant activity, anti-cancer actions, cardiovascular protection, and their most publicized use today, suppression of the vasomotor effects of menopause.

Prostate Health
Another interesting area of isoflavone intervention is in the treatment of prostate enlargement. Current modern treatment choices include

surgery or drugs. The drugs used today are either Alpha-1 blockers, which bind to specific receptors and cause the stroma (the framework of connective and muscle tissue) to relax, or 5a-reductase inhibitors, which block testosterone's conversion to dihydrotestosterone, decreasing an androgenic stimulus which causes the prostate to swell.

The current complementary medicine treatment for prostate enlargement, commonly referred to as benign prostate hyperplasia, is Saw Palmetto, which is a natural 5α-reductase inhibitor. However, etiological findings show men who consume large amounts of isoflavones in their diets maintain prostate function. For example, in countries that consume large quantities of legumes, prostate health is the norm. Prostate health is eight times higher in Japanese men than in American men. This link has been published in the *British Journal of Urology*, *Lancet*, and the *Medical Journal of Australia*.

The mechanism by which isoflavones positively affect prostate health is that, following consumption, isoflavones actively concentrate in prostate gland. Once localized, they exert a dual action to modulate mechanisms that regulate prostate health. They inhibit 5α reductase activity in ducts of glands, and they inhibit the enzymes that encourage cell proliferation in the stroma.

Modern Day Uses:
Menopause – Red Clover has been shown to reduce the two most common complaints of menopause, night sweats and hot flashes. It may also be valuable to maintain the elasticity of arteries and lower cholesterol, reducing the risk of coronary heart disease.

In addition to its most modern use, menopause, Red Clover may have a place in the treatment of begin prostate hyperplasia, and should not be completely discounted for some of its traditional uses, either alone or in combination with other herbs. These historic uses include cancer, as a general tonic, a blood cleanser, and to ameliorate spasms associated with asthma and bronchitis.

Dose:
The most clinically studied Red Clover preparation is one that is

standardized to contain 40 mg of the four primary isoflavone constituents, Genistein (4 mg), Daidzein (3.5 mg), Formononetin (8 mg), and Biochanin (24.5 mg). At this standardization level, taking just one tablet daily is equivalent to what the typical vegetarian or Japanese diet would provide by consuming legumes.

For more traditional preparations or herbal combination complexes, follow label directions.

Cautions:

If using a stand alone standardized extract, at the 40 mg isoflavone level, you are basically in the food range, and therefore it is no more harmful than eating a high legume diet. I would recommend not using Red Clover during pregnancy, and isoflavones are secreted in breast milk, so I would not exceed 40 mg during lactation.

No toxicity is associated with the use of even the highly standardized products as some Japanese, Korean, and vegetarian communities have been known to consume up to 100 mg of estrogenic isoflavones in their daily diets. However, if you are on any type of hormonal therapy, including birth control pills, care should be exercised in supplementing with estrogenic isoflavones. Phenolic estrogens can displace steroidal estrogens, which is a good thing if you are trying to prevent certain kinds of cancer such as breast cancer, but might complicate birth control. In the later case, consult with your health care professional.

Red Clover naturally contains coumarin and some coumarin-type phytochemicals. Therefore if you are taking anticoagulants or antiplatelet drugs like aspirin, you should monitor yourself more closely for enhanced risk of bleeding. You might be more susceptible. If this is the case, your physician may want to down-regulate your medication.

And lastly, since infertility disorders have been reported in grazing cattle, this is one of your natural medicines that you definitely want to keep away from the herd.

References:
See General Resources

Budbari, S, et al, eds. *The Merck Index*. 11ᵗʰ edition. Rathway, NJ. Merck & Co. 1989
Clarke, R, et al. "Estrogens, Phytoestrogens, and Breast Cancer." *Adv Experiment Med Biol*. 1996; 401:63-85

Knight, D, et al. "The Effects of Promensil™, an Isoflavone Extract, on Menopausal Symptoms." *Climacteric*. 1999; 2:79-84

Milsicek, R. "Interaction of Naturally Occurring Nonsteroidal Estrogens with Expressed Recombinant Human Estrogen Receptor." *Journal of Steroidal Biochemistry and Molecular Biology*. 1994; 49:153-160

Miodini, P, et al. "The Two Phyto-Estrogens Genistein and Quercetin Exert Different Effects on Estrogen Receptor Function." *Br J* Cancer 1999; 80:1150-5

Nachtigall, L, et al. "Nonprescription Alternatives to Hormone Replacement Therapy." *The Female Patient*. 1999; June. 24

Nestel, P, et al. "Isoflavones From Red Clover Improve Systemic Compliance But Not Plasma Lipids in Menopausal Women." *Journal of Clinical Endocrinology and Metabolism*. 1999; 84:895-98

Promensil Technical and Safety Information Bulletin. Stamford, CT. Novagen, Inc. 1998

Rhodiola

(Rhodiola rosea)

Other Common Names:
Golden Root, Rosavin, Rose Root, Rose Wort

Background:
Up until fairly recently, this plant was practically unknown in the United States. And, now this Russian secret has become one of my personal favorites. Golden Root is indigenous to the Golden Circle region of eastern Siberia. It grows at altitudes of 11,000 to 18,000 feet above sea level. Its yellow flowers smell like roses, hence the name "rosea." This wonderful botanical is so new to us that I am not sure which of its most used names is going to become the common one, Rhodiola or Golden Root. Therefore, to be politically correct, I am going to use both.

The legend of Golden Root's health and longevity benefits has been passed from generation to generation for 3,000 years. It is said that people who drink Rhodiola tea will live to be over 100 years old. It is one of the common supplements used by the famous Georgian people, who do live over a 100 years. They use it to increase physical endurance, and to fight depression and fatigue. Chinese Emperors sought the Golden Root to treat a variety of diseases. Mongolian doctors prescribed an extract of Golden Root to treat tuberculosis and cancer. In addition, a Russian botanist discovered that Golden Root increased sexual potency, which validates a Siberian folk tradition of giving the plant extract to couples prior to marriage to help ensure the birth of healthy children.

In 1947, a Soviet scientist from the Far-East Academy of Sciences reported that several plants indigenous to Siberia helped increase the body's ability to handle stress. In 1958, Dr. I Brekhman of the USSR coined the term, "adaptogen," and introduced the concept of natural bioactive compounds having the ability to increase a human's resistance to different stress-related disorders. Said another way, an adaptogen is something that can increase the body's general adaptive strength.

Of course, most of the active research on adaptogens targeted Siberian Ginseng (Eleutherococcus). However, a small group at the Russian Academy of Sciences directed their research to Rhodiola rosea. In 1961, decent amounts of wild Rhodiola were found growing at lower elevations, making it more available for research. In the early 1990s, because of the Soviet breakup, many years of research was released to the rest of the world.

The healing properties of Golden Root are quite a list. The following are a few of the human afflictions that the plant extract has been used and clinically validated for:

> ➢ Increased attention span and memory
> ➢ Up-regulation of vitality and stress handling capability
> ➢ Cardio-protective outcomes
> ➢ Maintenance of focus over long periods of work
> ➢ Anti-tumor activity
> ➢ Reduction of blood sugar
> ➢ Prevention of altitude sickness
> ➢ Anti-allergy actions
> ➢ Anti-depressant activity

Science:

Standardization

The major phytochemicals found in Rhodiola rosea include beta sistosterol, cinnamic alcohol, rhodiolon, tyrasol, gallic acid, and other phenolic compounds. Those constituents exerting the highest biological activity include the phenylproponoids, salidrozid, rosin, rosarin, and rosavin. Many extracts are standardized to salidroside or total polyphenols, but this could be problematic.

Botanists have identified 20 species of Rhodiola, with only a few undergoing serious scientific study. They all contain salidrozid, as do White Willow Bark, Blueberry, Cranberry, and Rhododendron. Only R. rosea, the most biologically active and clinically tested species, contains rosavin. Therefore, an extract should be standardized to rosavin. This ensures that you are getting R. rosea and prevents any possible adulteration, as rosavin can be the only true identification marker. The extract that I have personally used is standardized to a minimum of .8% rosavin.

Rhodiola as an adaptogen and cardioprotective agent

Adaptogens are tonics; they tone the organism by simultaneously up and down-regulating body systems as needed. The end result is a host that can better resist the ravages of stress. What it looks like is an improved physical work capacity (stamina and endurance), improved mental capacity, and more rapid recovery from work and fatigue.

Some of the mechanisms by which Rhodiola rosea works for us are:

> ➤ Regulation of the adrenal hormones involved in the fight, flight, fright response (catecholamines).
> ➤ Dampening of potentially harmful adrenal hormones like cortisol that is released when the body is stressed, while enhancing the hypothalamus' release of stress fighting hormones like ACTH (adrenocorticotropic hormone).
> ➤ Enhanced utilization of oxygen and fats in the production of energy.

Animal studies have shown Rhodiola to protect the heart against known arrhythmic stressors, in addition to having a cholesterol lowering effect. Additionally, it has been shown to be a potent antioxidant. Antioxidants have been shown to slow hardening of the arteries.

Rhodiola and depression

Rhodiola has been shown to enhance the level of serotonin, dopamine and nor-epinephrine, three brain neurotransmitters that need to be present in sufficient quantities to maintain a healthy mood. In fact, all the antidepressant drugs on the market today address up-regulating these substances.

5-hydroxytryptophan (5-HTP), which is synthesized from the amino acid tryptophan, is a precursor to serotonin. Monoamine oxidase (MAO) and catechol-o-methyltransferase (COMT) are enzymes that degrade brain neurotransmitters. After many years of research, Russian scientists have demonstrated that Rhodiola's role in preventing or treating depression lies in its ability to enhance the transport of tryptophan and 5HTP into the brain, and its inhibitory effect on MAO and COMT.

In Russia, Rhodiola rosea has been used as an adjunct to conventional drug therapy. Their experience is that the patients' general activity, intellectual and physical productivity increased while untoward effects of the drugs decreased. Closer to home, those managing their mood with St. John's Wort who still have room for improvement should consider adding Rhodiola.

As a side note on COMT inhibition, I should mention that reduced levels of dopamine in the brain is consistent with Parkinson's disease. This degenerative disorder is treated with drugs like levodopa that increase brain dopamine. There is a new class of drugs being developed that are COMT inhibitors. They will be used with levodopa, reducing its breakdown before it enters the brain, thereby enhancing its effect by increasing its availability to the brain. This class of drugs will also generate candidates used to treat depression.

Rhodiola rosea and cancer

Rhodiola has been shown to increase an organism's resistance to tumor formation and growth. In animal experiments, Rhodiola significantly inhibited the formation and growth of experimental cancers, decreased their metastastases (spread), and prolonged the life expectancy of the host. It was also shown to stimulate liver generation, an important function during cancer therapy. In human studies, when Rhodiola was given to patients with bladder cancer, they experienced improvement in immune function and a decrease in the frequency of relapse.

The mechanism by Rhodiola rosea exerts these effects is not clear. However, it is believed that its powerful antioxidant activity protects against lipid peroxidation, a mechanism that leads to pathological damage and mutations. There is also speculation that it inhibits colony-forming activity, an important mechanism in tumor formation.

Rhodiola rosea and weight management

Stored body fat is a difficult thing to rid oneself of. Anyone embarking on the diet and exercise roller coaster can relate to this stubborn process. Stored fat can be mobilized by the action of a special enzyme known as "hormone sensitive lipase." For many years, researchers have been searching for natural substances to activate cellular lipolysis. Remarkably, this property was discovered in Rhodiola thirty years ago and concealed from the West until recently. Research over this thirty-year period on both healthy volunteers and obese patients shows that the administration of Rhodiola specifically mobilizes fat from its fat warehouses.

The mechanism by which Rhodiola rosea administration facilitates stored fat breakdown is based on its ability to activate something called adenosine 3c,5c-cyclic monophosphate (cAMP). cAMP acts as a messenger in very complicated cellular metabolism. However, by way of simplification, during aerobic exercise, a mechanism by which your body taps into fat stores to be burned for fuel involves cAMP activation. What seems to be the beauty of Rhodiola is that this activation takes place early, enabling more fat to be released for immediate energy use with less effort.

The Soviets have conducted studies to validate Rhodiola's effects on fat mobilization. As much as I try to avoid boring study details, a few of these trials bear mentioning.

Study 1: A group of 121 healthy subjects were measured for their level of fatty acids in serum at rest and after one hour of bicycle exercise. The group was divided in half, one set of volunteers receiving Rhodiola, the other a placebo. At rest, serum fatty acids did not go up appreciably, although the Rhodiola group did show a 6% increase over the control group.

After 60 minutes of exercise, the results were extremely impressive. Serum fatty acid levels increased in both groups, as expected, but the Rhodiola group showed a 44% increase over the control group.

These results provided clear evidence that Rhodiola coupled with exercise can be a powerful tool in activating stored fat for fuel, leading to safe weight reduction. It should however be noted that these results were reproducible with species of Rhodiola that did not contain rosavin.

Study 2: Patients were divided into two groups, one group received Rhodiola, the other a placebo. Samples of blood serum were taken after 30 minutes of normal walking. Again, as in the previous study, serum levels of fatty acids were higher in the Rhodiola group, this time by 17%.

Study 3: Two groups of obese patients were instructed to eat as they pleased but were required to walk for 30-40 minutes after each meal. Their diet included junk foods like chips, sweets and pizza. One group took 100 mg of Rhodiola before each meal; the other did not. At the end of three months, both groups were evaluated for weight loss, and both groups did indeed lose weight (walking works). However, the Rhodiola groups lost 11% of their body weight, while the control group only lost 4%.

Modern Day Uses:

The list of uses for an adaptogen herb can be endless. Ginseng is a perfect example. Rhodiola rosea, however, seems to be more than just an adaptogen. Following is a list of conditions and benefits that the Golden Root might be considered for:

> General health and a feeling of well-being
> Stress support
> Depression
> Cardiovascular disease
> General immunity
> Cancer
> Physical performance
> Mental performance
> Parkinson's disease
> Diabetic support
> Weight loss

➤ Sexual performance
➤ Acute mountain sickness

What piqued my interest in Rhodiola was that it had been studied for its cardiopulmonary benefits at high altitudes. When I uncovered this fact, I was in the process of preparing myself for a mountaineering trip in the Andes. I was able to procure some raw material called Rosavin™ and like a good pharmacist, punched my own capsules. I began taking 100 mg three times daily.

I felt that it shortened my recovery time after prolonged workouts and reduced my muscle trauma after exhaustive exercise. After using the extract for a relatively short period of time, I was able to trim minutes off my five mile hill run. I also felt that it made a significant contribution to a reduction in my body fat. I took the product to South America with me and felt that it benefited me on my climb. Needless to say, I became a believer, and have become an advocate of Golden Root. It has become my personal favorite adaptogenic supplement, replacing Ginseng.

Dose:
Using an extract standardized to rosavin, take 100 mg 2 to 3 times daily before meals.

Cautions:
Golden root has proven itself to be an extremely safe herb, with no known contraindications or ill effects. Its safety record is backed by extensive Russian work, but this wonderful botanical medicine has not been widely used in the United States yet.

References:
See General Resources

Bocharova, O, et al. "The Effects of Rhodiola Rosea Extract on the Incidence of Recurrences Bladder Cancer." *Urol Nefrol*. 1995; 2:46-7

Bogdshin, I, et al. "The Effect of Rhodiola Extract on the Cytotoxic Activity of the Natural Killer Cells of the Liver, Spleen, Lungs, and Gut in Rat After Partial Hepatectomy." *Experimental Medicine*. 1990; 110:409-11

Dementyeva, L, et al. "The Study of the Influence of Rhodiola Rosea Extract on the Growth of Tumors in Experiment." *Bul Sib Dep of the Academy of Sciences/USSR*. 1983, No. 6

Khushbatove, Z, et al. "Study of the Hypolipidemic Properties of Plymer Proanthocyanidins form Plants Used in Folk Medicine." *Pharmaceutical Journal*. 1989; 23:1111-15

Lishmanov, I, et al. "The Anti- arrhythmia Effect of Rhodiola Rosea and its Possible Mechanism." *Biull Eksp Biol Med*. 1993; 116:175-6

Maimeskulova, L, et al. "The Participation of the MU, Delta and Kappa-opiod Receptors in the Realization of the Anti- arrhythmia Effect of Rhodiola Rosea." *Eksp KlinFarmakol*. 1997; 60:38-9

Maslova, L, et al. "The Cardioprotective and Antiadrenergic Activity of an Extract of Rhodiola Rosea in Stress." *Eksp KlinFarmakol*. 1994; 57:61-3

Ramazanov, Z, et al. *The Powerful New Ginseng Alternative*. New York, NY. Kensington Publishing Co. 1999

Ramazanov, Zakir. Personal Communiqué. Dec. 1999, April 2000, October 2000.

Ramazanov, Z, et al. *Effective Natural Stress and Weight Management Using Rhodiola Rosea and Rhododendron Caucasicum*. East Canaan, CT. ATN/Safe Goods Publishing. 1999

Saratikov, A, et al. "Rhodiola Rosea as a Valuable Medicinal Plant." *Tomsk*. 1987; 252

Udintzev, S, et al. "The Role of Humoral Factors of Regenerating Liver in the Development of Experimental Tumors and the Effect of Rhodiola Rosea Extract on the Process." *Neoplasma*. 1991; 38:323-332

Zhang, Z, et al. "Effect of Rhodiola on Preventing High Altitude Reactions: A Comparison of Cardiopulmonary Function in Villagers at Different Altitude Areas." *Journal of Chinese Materia Medica*. 1989; 14:47-50

Zhang, Z, et al. "Electron Microspopic Observation of the Effects of Rhodiola in Preventing Damage of the Rat Viscera by a Hypoxic High Altitude Environment." *Chung Kuo Chung Yao Tsa Chih*. 1990; 3:177-81

Saw Palmetto

(Serenoa repens)

Other Common Names:

Sabal, Sabal serrulata, Serenoa serrulata, American Dwarf Palm Tree, Cabbage Palm, Fan Palm, Dwarf Palmetto

Background:

Saw Palmetto is a small palm tree native to the North American East Coast from South Carolina to Florida and west to Texas. Native Americans used its berries as both a food and a medicine. Legend has it that when our early settlers observed animals grow "sleek and fat" upon feeding on the berries, they tried them and attributed medicinal properties to them. Then, they proceeded to use the leaves for making brooms. Apparently not all colonials were fast reactors.

It was not until the 1870s that Saw Palmetto acquired some popularity, following a series of medical publications suggesting diuretic, sedative, and anticatarrhal properties. Catarrh is an old term referring to the inflammation of mucous membranes with increased flow of mucus or exudate.

The Eclectic's wasted organs

At the end of the 19th century, Saw Palmetto gained a clinical reputation in medicine, particularly in the Eclectic school, a now defunct system of medicine that advocated use of indigenous plants to effect specific cures of certain signs and symptoms. *King's American Dispensary* was the publication that represented a compilation of the Eclectics' experiential knowledge and lists the following uses for Saw Palmetto: an expectorant for various coughs, laryngitis, asthma, and a digestive for appetite. It also refers to Saw Palmetto's usefulness for the enlargement of "wasted organs," namely breasts, ovaries and testicles. I'm not sure what they meant by "wasted," but I am sure that if my physician referred to one of my organs as being "wasted," I would not consider it good news.

Saw Palmetto's early official drug status

King's goes on to state that "long-continued use of it (Saw Palmetto) is said to slowly and surely cause mammae to enlarge." Saw Palmetto was also referred to in the 23rd edition of the *United States Dispensatory*, 45 years later, as having the ability to allay the symptoms of "the enlarged prostate of old men." The enthusiasm generated by Saw Palmetto led to the marketing of Palmetto Wine. In those days, it was believed that the berries possessed infection-controlling effects, and in this way, controlled prostate problems. However, today we better understand the complex mechanisms by which the herb has gained its reputation.

Saw Palmetto berries were actually an official drug in the *United Sates Pharmacopoeia* from 1906 to 1916. The accepted indications included chronic and sub-acute cystitis, chronic bronchitis, laryngitis, catarrh that accompanies asthma, and enlarged prostate. It was also an official drug in the *National Formulary* from 1926-1950. Over the early part of these years, as it was also thought to increase sperm production and sex drive in men, it became a popular tonic for men.

However, over its history, as briefly referred to above, Saw Palmetto has not always been just for men. For women, it has been used to treat infertility, increase lactation, allay painful periods, and as a general tonic for ovarian function. It has also been used as a general nutritive to increase fat, muscle and strength. It has been a mild sedative for the nervous system, an anti-inflammatory, appetite stimulant, and has been used to treat digestive troubles and thyroid deficiency.

Science:

It is the berries of Saw Palmetto that are harvested for its health benefits. They contain nine fatty acids, three steroids, diterpenes, triterpenes, a sesquiterpene, and five alcohols. It is generally recognized that it is the fatty acids that are key to Saw Palmetto's hormone modulating activity, and concentrated standardized extracts are now available for that purpose.

Even though Saw Palmetto is a native American plant, almost all the clinical research initiated on it has come from Germany, France, and

Italy. This research has lead to the conclusions that Saw Palmetto is definitely anti-androgenic, anti-exudative, and is a 5-alpha reductase inhibitor.

Saw Palmetto and the benign prostatic hyperplasia (BPH) connection

BHP is believed to be caused by an accumulation of testosterone in the prostate. This surplus testosterone is then converted to the more potent dihydrotestosterone, which then causes cells to multiply excessively, eventually causing the prostate to enlarge. The fatty acid constituents of Saw Palmetto berries prevent the conversion of testosterone to dihydrotestosterone by inhibiting the rate-limiting enzyme, 5-alpha reductase. But that's not all. These fatty substances also block dihydrotestosterone's ability to bind to its receptor sites, thereby increasing its breakdown and excretion.

There's more. In addition to Saw Palmetto's anti-androgen activity, it also has anti-estrogen activity. This is significant because estrogen inhibits the elimination of dihydrotestosterone, the very stuff we're trying to get rid of. It is also important to note that both the anti-androgen and anti-estrogen effects are localized. That is, Saw Palmetto does not exert systemic hormonal changes.

Besides Saw Palmetto's direct effect on the prostate, it has two additional actions of interest. Constituents of the berries are anti-inflammatory. They inhibit the enzymes cyclo-oxygenase and 5-lipoxygenase, thereby reducing levels of inflammatory prostaglandins and leukotrienes. Additionally, Saw Palmetto's polysaccharides have immune stimulating activity, which is probably why early uses included cystitis.

Modern Day Uses:

First and foremost, Saw Palmetto is indicated to relieve the symptoms of benign prostatic hyperplasia (BPH). The symptoms include, but are not limited to, obstruction of the bladder outlet, interrupted sleep patterns (secondary to nocturia), frequent urge to urinate, incomplete bladder emptying, occasional burning sensation with urination, frequent dribbling, urine retention, and hesitancy and intermittency of the urinary stream.

Natural actually performed better than synthetic
Saw Palmetto has actually outperformed synthetic drugs in clinical studies. In one study, the researchers concluded that Saw Palmetto offered superior symptomatic relief to the drug finasteride, as defined by the most common clinical tests. It was concluded that Saw Palmetto improves quality of life and has a "practically negligible side effect risk." And keep in mind that Saw Palmetto, in contrast to finasteride, inhibits the binding of DHT to its receptor and has, as well, some anti-estrogen effects. This means that it actually has a greater spectrum of action.

In a review of 18 controlled clinical studies, *JAMA* (Journal of the American Medical Association) authors concluded that Saw Palmetto was more effective than placebo, and just as effective as the standard drug finasteride, in relieving the symptoms of moderate BPH. Compared to finasteride, Saw Palmetto appears to have a better track record, helping nearly 90% of patients compared to less than 50% helped by finasteride. And, Saw Palmetto works faster, within four to six weeks compared to one year.

A treatment for male baldness?
Males born without 5-alpha reductase never suffer male pattern baldness, BPH, or prostate cancer. Research has determined that the balding scalp of men contains increased amounts of dihydrotestosterone, compared to hairy scalps. Well, let's go out on a limb here. If you block the dihydrotestosterone with a 5-alpha reductase inhibitor, you can stop hair loss and/or grow hair back.

Well, Merck & Co., the makers of Proscar® (finasteride), gave it a go. The results were that 66% of the men receiving 1 mg of finasteride daily (compared to the 5 mg dose for BPH) for two years grew hair, compared with 7% of those given placebo. What fascinated me was how the 7% who didn't get the drug grew hair. Nevertheless, even though withdrawal of the drug leads to reversal of the effects within 12 months, you cannot deny that the finasteride increased hair count. The down side is the adverse-effect profile of the drug, which includes decreased libido, erectile dysfunction, and ejaculation disorder. Is baldness sounding better? I would try Saw Palmetto.

Dose:

In order to achieve maximum benefits for BPH, use a concentrated Saw Palmetto extract, standardized to 85%-95% fatty acids. Take 160 mg twice daily. You cannot achieve an active compound dose with other preparations. The berries themselves only contain about 1.5% fatty acids. So, you can see, if you do the math, that you would have to take 40 capsules a day of 500 mg crude berries to get the same amount of actives. Recent research has elucidated that a once daily, 320 mg dose may be equally effective.

Since the commercial raw material, standardized to 85% to 95% fatty acids, only comes in an oil, a more practical alternative is to use a powdered extract which is standardized to about 25% fatty acids. Taking 600 mg twice daily would then impart the same health benefits. And, if you find a product that claims to be standardized to 85% to 95%, and it is either in a hard-gel capsule or a tablet, ask how they do that. Unless the manufacturer has invented new science, which is possible, that product may be improperly labeled.

Cautions:

Since the Seminole Indians used Saw Palmetto as a food source, one has to believe that this is a pretty safe herb. No side effects have been attributed to Saw Palmetto, nor are there known interactions with conventional drugs. Furthermore, it does not interfere with PSA testing (prostate specific antigen is used as a marker in diagnosing prostate cancer).

Since the symptoms of BPH are identical to those of prostate cancer, I strongly discourage self-diagnosis. BPH should be diagnosed by a physician! No exceptions!

References:
See General Resources

Bach, D. and Ebeling, L. "Long-term Drug Treatment of Benign Prostatic Hyperplasia." *Phytomedicine*. 1996. 3:105-111

Bach, D., et al. "Phytopharmaceutical and Synthetic Agents in the Treatment of Benign Prostatic Hyperplasia (BHP)." *Phytomedicine* 1997. ¾:309-313

Bayne, C, et al. "Serenoa repens: A 5-Alpha-Reductase Types I and II Inhibitor- New Evidence in a Coculture Model of BPH." *Prostate*. 1999; 40:232-41

Braeckman, J. "The Extract of Serenoa repens in the Treatment of BPH: A Multicenter Open Study." *Current Therapeutic Research*. 1994. 55:776-85

Carraro, J., et al. "Comparison of the Phytotherapy with Finasteride in the Treatment of Benign Prostate Hyperplasia: A Randomized International Study of 1098 Patients." *Prostate*. 1996. 29:231-240

Casarosa, C., et al. "Lack of Effects of a Lyposterolic Extract of Serenoa repens on Plasma Levels of Testosterone, FSH, and LH." *Clin Ther*. 1988. 10:585-8

Crooms, E, and Walker, L. "Botanicals in the Pharmacy: New Life for Old Remedies." *Drug Topics*. Continuing Education. Nov 1995

Duke, J. *The Green Pharmacy*. Emmaus, PA, Rodale Press. 1997

Felter, H and Lloyd, J. *King's American Dispensatory* 1898. Portland, OR. Eclectic Medical Publications 1983

O'Hara, M, et al. "A Review of 12 Commonly Used Medicinal Herbs." *Arch Fam Med*. 1998; 7:523-536

Stepanov, V, et al. "Efficacy and Tolerability of the Lipidosterolic Extract of Serenoa repens in Benign Prostatic Hyperplasia: A Double Blind Comparison of Two Dosage Forms." *Advances Therapy*. 1999; 16:231-41

Wilt, T. et al. "Saw Palmetto Extracts for Treatment of BPH: A Systematic Review. *JAMA* 1998. 280 (18):1604-1609

Scullcap

(Scutellaria lateriflora, Scutellaria spp.)

Other Common Names:
Mad-Dog Scullcap, Mad Dogweed, Madweed, Mad Dog, Helmet Flower, Pimpernel, Hood Wort, Hooded Willow Herb, Quaker's Bonnet, Greater Scullcap

Background:
This perennial member of the mint family numbers over 300 species, 113 of which grow in the Americas. Of all of them, S. lateriflora, or Common Scullcap, is the best known.

As evidenced by many of Scullcap's common names, this plant has history of treating rabies. In fact, in the late 18th century, a Dr. Lawrence Van Derveer of Roysfield, New Jersey, made a career out of treating rabies, and he did it with Scullcap. He is said to have treated 400 cases of rabies, only losing two patients. I think that is a lot of cases of rabies for one town. Perhaps they should have renamed it Mad Dog, New Jersey.

Traditionally, Scullcap leaf has been used as a nerve tonic and for nerve conditions such as anxiety, neuralgia, insomnia, and epilepsy. It was also considered a treatment for St. Vitus's Dance, which is characterized by irregular, spasmodic, involuntary movements of the limbs or facial muscles, often accompanied by hypotonia (extreme muscle tension).

Scullcap , an official drug of the 1860 *United States Pharmacopoeia*, was dropped in 1870, picked up again in 1880, and dropped in 1900. It managed to stay in the *National Formulary* (a book of standards used by the American Pharmaceutical Association now taken over by the *U.S. Pharmacopoeia*) until 1947.

Science:
Scullcap is an herbal that has been beat up a little. One author wrote

that calling Scullcap a useful tranquilizing herb says much about the gullibility of human beings. However, many of the classic herbal texts, which he likes to reference, refer to Scullcap for its tonic, nervine and antispasmodic actions. He calls it worthless inactive plant material. I say, you can't have it both ways.

Other texts warn of the use of Scullcap with other herbs and drugs that have sedative properties. Why would this be necessary for inactive plant material? It is a given that despite the traditional uses of Scullcap as a sedative and anticonvulsant, ittle scientific data supports these uses, and little information has been elucidated regarding its chemistry. However, can you discount centuries of folk use? One of the few studies done on Scullcap did support its use as a mild sedative, so let's give it the benefit of the doubt and agree that this plant is a candidate for more studies.

It should be noted that the root of a Chinese species of Scullcap is being studied, but for its activity on microbes, blood pressure, inflammation, cancer, and liver disease.

Modern Day Uses:
The famous herbalist Dr. John Christopher was fond of Scullcap. He found it calming when nervousness resulted from worry, conflict, and disturbances of digestion and circulation. He found it useful to treat restlessness and often combined it with other herbs for insomnia.

Dose:
The usual dose is 1-2 capsules up to three times daily, or as recommended by the manufacturer.

Cautions:
None known. How could worthless inactive plant material have side effects?

References:

See General Resources

Chung, C, et al. "Pharmacological Effects of Methanolic Extract From the Root of Scutellaria Baicalensis and Its Flavonoids on Human Fibroblast." *Planta Med.* 1995; 61:150-53

Foster, S. "Scullcap: An Herbal Enigma." *The Business of Herbs.* 1996; 5/6:14-16

Goldberg, V, et al. ""Dry Extract of Scutellaria Baicalensis as a Hemostimulant in Antineoplastic Chemotherapy in Patients with Lung Cancer." *Eksp Klin Farmakol.* 1997; 60:28-30

Kubo, M, et al. "Studies on Scutellariae Radix. Part II: The Antibacterial Substance." *Planta Med.* 1981; 43:194-201

St. John's Wort

(Hypericum perforatum)

Other Common Names:

John's Wort, Klamath Weed, Amber Touch-And-Heal, Goatweed, Rosin Rose, Millepertuis, Amber, Devil's Scourge, God's Wonder Plant, Grace Of God, Witches' Herb

Background:

St. John's Wort is an aromatic perennial that yields a golden yellow flower. It is native to Europe but is now found throughout the U.S., growing exceptionally well in Northern California, and Southern Oregon. It is an aggressive weed and grows along roadsides and meadows in dry gravelly ground. The plant usually grows between 1 and 2 feet in height, unless you're on my Pacific coast where it has been know to get up to five feet. This would explain why ranchers, who considered it a nuisance, managed to reduce it to one percent of its original wild population. That is until the boom of the 90s.

The plant is a little temperamental when it comes to harvesting. It is generally harvested between July and August. Once picked, it must be immediately dried. If this is not done, it will lose its medicinal potency. An unusual phenomenon occurs during the medicinal preparation of this plant, in that a green plant with a yellow flower ends up being a blood red extract, like magic.

Some believe that St. John's Wort takes its common name from the Knights of St. John of Jerusalem, who used it to treat wounds on Crusade battlefields. Others believe that it got its common name from the red extract that symbolizes the blood of St. John the Baptist. Some believe the name comes from the medieval belief that if you slept with a piece of plant under your pillow, St. John would come into your dream and grant you another year of life with his blessings. While still others say it got its name because it blooms right around St. John's Day (June 24), the anniversary of the day St. John the Baptist was beheaded.

The medicinal history of St. John's Wort, like that of so many of today's top herbs, goes back to ancient Greece, where Hippocrates, Dioscorides, and Pliny used it for sciatica, as a diuretic, for menstrual problems, external wounds, burns, and poisonous reptile bites. Its genus name, *Hypericum*, comes from the Greek meaning "over an apparition," or to overcome a ghost. This is a reference to St. John's reputation as driving a force to expel evil spirits. St. John's Wort was administered to the insane in an effort to dispel their demons.

Wound healing and neurological effects were described by Galen (130-200 AD), and repeated throughout the Middle Ages. Sixteenth century British herbalist, John Gerard praised the extract as a most precious remedy for deep wounds. Traditionally, St. John's Wort has been used as an anti-inflammatory agent, a topical treatment for wounds, scabies, hemorrhoids, and a host of other ailments including anxiety, nerve pain, and sedation, bronchitis, cancer, gastritis, hypothyroidism, kidney disorders, and neuralgia. Today, it is not used much for most of these actions, but the interest it has sparked is for its marked influence on depression.

Paracelsus (1493–1541) was the first physician to use Hypericum to treat depression, melancholy and related states. Since then, it has slowly built a reputation as a mood altering substance. Today, the clinical evidence is overwhelming in favor of Hypericum extract as a virtually risk free antidepressant for the treatment of mild to moderate depression.

Who would have thought that Hugh and Barbara were capable of changing the course of herbal history. In June of 1997, on their magazine program, 20/20, they reintroduced St. John's Wort to the masses. Within weeks, there wasn't a kilogram of raw material to be had anywhere in the country, and perhaps the world. In a well-balanced report, based on good science, St. John's Wort was presented as a viable alternative to standard antidepressant drugs.

Science:
The anthraquinone derivative, hypericin, is the best known ingredient in St. John's Wort. We used to think it was the plant's active ingredient

responsible for its antidepressant activity. Other components include pseudohypericin, Hyperforin, flavonoids, phenolic carboxylic acids, and essential oils. St. John's Wort also contains about 10% tannin. This may contribute to its wound healing effects, through tannin's astringent and protein precipitation actions.

Following the lead of the Germans, St. John's Wort preparations are generally standardized to hypericin, the phytochemical believed to have been its primary active. Unfortunately, recent research has concluded that hypericin may not be responsible for the activity of the extract. The active ingredient, as so often in plants, is likely to be not singular, but a symphonic effort among ingredients, with a new kid on the block called Hyperforin now thought to be the conductor. Even though in this country hypericin is still used a marker, in Germany, products are no longer allowed to be labeled based on hypericin content.

Antidepressant
A 1996 meta-analysis of 23 controlled clinical trials verified that St. John's Wort was an effective treatment for mild to moderate depression. Eight studies that compared it to low dose tricyclic antidepressants showed St. John's Wort to be of equivalent efficacy, with significantly fewer side effects. Depression indicators used included feelings of sadness, hopelessness, helplessness, uselessness, fear, and sleep disorders.

More and more studies are coming out on a regular basis. While previous clinical data was available on head to head comparisons between St. John's Wort and placebos, and St. John's Wort and tricyclic antidepressants, now favorable reports are coming in comparing St. John's Wort and SSRIs (selective serotonin re-uptake inhibitors…like Prozac®), even in the elderly.

We are currently unclear what the actives are and what their mechanisms could be. The original theoretical mechanism responsible for the antidepressant effect of Hypericum was believed to be associated with monoamine oxidase (MAO) inhibition. MAO is the enzyme that degrades synaptic catacholamine neurotransmitters. However, we soon learned that the level of MAO inhibition found in the plant is not enough to account for its clinical activity. The next theory suggested that hypericin extract acted by impairing the reuptake of serotonin. This is the same mechanism of action that Prozac® exerts. However, now hypericin is no longer considered to be the significant active.

Recent attention, as mentioned above, has gone to Hyperforin. A recent study using rat models of "learned helplessness," (I can relate to these rats; I used to cook before I got married) and "learned behavioral despair" were used to test Hyperforin. The results showed significant inhibition of various reuptakes, any of which alone would account for the extract's antidepressant activity. The neurotransmitters included norepinephrine, dopamine, GABA, and serotonin. Once again, MAO inhibitory activity was insignificant. It should be noted that there is no drug available that can affect all of these uptake systems, making St. John's Wort a unique antidepressant.

Antiviral and antibacterial
Hypericin is being evaluated as a treatment against human immunodeficiency virus (HIV), based on its action against retroviruses.

Hypericin and pseudohypericin are effective against a wide spectrum of viruses including influenza A and B, herpes simplex 1 and 2, sindbis (malaria-like), polio, and hepatitis. The mechanism by which these phytochemicals exert their antiviral effects remain a mystery. We know it has nothing to do with transcription, translation, or protein transport.

Extracts of St. John's Wort are also effective against bacteria. They are active against both gram-positive and gram-negative strains. Some of the organisms against which it has been found effective include Staphylococcus, Streptococcus, Proteus, Pseudomonas, and E Coli.

Modern Day Uses:
For those seeking a natural alternative to prescription anti-depressant drugs, St. John's Wort may be an ideal treatment. But remember, this option is only for those with mild or moderate conditions. If you believe that you are more severely affected, please see a health profes-

sional. In Germany, physicians prescribe St. John's Wort four times more often than fluoxetine (Prozac®).

The symptoms of depression are listed below. Usually you are considered depressed if you have at least four symptoms and have had them for at least two weeks.

Psychological symptoms
> ➢ Anxiety
> ➢ Agitation
> ➢ Feelings of hopelessness
> ➢ Feelings of worthlessness
> ➢ Feelings of excessive guilt
> ➢ Restlessness
> ➢ Indecisiveness
> ➢ Apathy
> ➢ Loss of drive
> ➢ Melancholy
> ➢ Low self esteem
> ➢ Loss of interest
> ➢ Loss of pleasure

Physical symptoms
> ➢ Fatigue
> ➢ Energy loss
> ➢ Change in appetite
> ➢ Sexual difficulties
> ➢ Change in memory
> ➢ Poor concentration
> ➢ Chronic constipation
> ➢ Sleep habit changes
> ➢ Dry mouth
> ➢ Chest tightness (ruling out a physical cause)

Other uses for St. John's Wort include:

> ➢ Psychological and vegetative symptoms of menopause
> ➢ PMS
> ➢ Nervous disorders

> ➤ Mania
> ➤ Sleep
> ➤ Bed-wetting
> ➤ Childhood nightmares
> ➤ Nerve pain
> ➤ Unexplained fatigue
> ➤ Season Affective Disorder
> ➤ Fibromyalgia
> ➤ Migraines
> ➤ Sciatica
> ➤ Burning or tingling pain
> ➤ Pain associated with inflamed nerves (tooth socket pain, shingles, trigeminal neuralgia, fractures, surgical, injury from stabbing or burns, various traumas)

Topical uses (as an oil, tea, gel, cream, or tincture): antiseptic, wound healing, abrasions, burns, frostbite, insect bites, hemorrhoids, herpes lesions, muscular pain, sciatica, neuralgia.

Dose:

An effective regimen has been 300 mg of an extract, standardized to 0.3% hypericin, taken 3 times daily, and it is not unreasonable to double this dose if necessary. This range has been effective because these extracts probably contain some unknown amount of Hyperforin. I think we will be seeing more products on the market with a guaranteed amount of Hyperforin. This may make the difference for those who tried St. John's Wort but were disappointed with the results. The products that had a high Hyperforin content may have been the products that were the most effective. Start looking for products standardized for Hyperforin.

As with prescription antidepressant medication, there is a several week lag between drug initiation and clinical efficacy. The key to antidepressant treatment, whether with pharmaceuticals or Nature, is patience. One must allow at least three weeks before evaluating results and considering a medication change.

Cautions:

With all the millions of doses of St. John's Wort consumed every year, it has become famous for is low incidence of adverse reactions. Occasional reports of mild gastrointestinal upset, dry mouth, nervousness, and skin rash have been reported.

St. John's Wort should not be taken with other SSRI (selective serotonin reuptake inhibitor) drugs. Doing so increases the risk of serotonin syndrome, which is caused by an overdose of serotonin. However, I recognize that many people are interested in using St. Johns Wort as a replacement for medications they are already on. In this case, St. John's Wort can be slowly introduced while your medication is slowly weaned down. Work with your healthcare professional. I am sure that you will not be the first person to have approached him or her with this request.

Many, less enlightened, like to drive fear into the souls of St. John's Wort users by telling them if they take the extract and go into the sun, they will be scorched. This is known as photosensitivity, and many drugs have this side effect. I believe this came to be when some hungry cows made pigs of themselves in a meadow covered with St. John's Wort. They did become photosensitive, but they were in such a good mooood, they didn't care.

Clinicians I have talked to, and whose lectures I have had the privilege to attend, claim they have never had an incident of photosensitivity in their practices. So, it is reasonable to say that unless you are going out grazing, there is little likelihood of becoming photosensitive with normal therapeutic doses of St. John's Wort. However, if you are taking large doses of St. John's Wort, first ask yourself why you are doing that, and then be aware of the possibility of sunburn. Incidentally, this would be a mute point if we all followed the advice of our dermatology experts and never stepped outdoors without first using sunscreen.

Women of child-bearing age should take note that there is speculation that St. John's Wort may decrease the effectiveness of birth control pills. If you think you had problems before.... I suggest an alternate contraceptive method. So far, this is just speculation and studies confirming this are yet to be done. However, you are forewarned.

On the other had, St. John's Wort may interfere with sperm motility. Therefore, couples experiencing fertility problems should avoid its use.

St. John's Wort may increase the pharmacokinetics of digoxin, a drug used for, among other things, congestive heart failure. This can result in a reduced blood level of the drug. Do not use concomitantly, without the advice of your healthcare professional.

While studies were being conducted using St. John's Wort in AIDS, it was discovered that when taken in combination with another AIDS drug, a protease inhibitor called indinavir, St. John's Wort substantially decreased indinavir's plasma concentrations. This has led to speculation that it may also interfere with drugs that are similarly metabolized. Birth control pills were one of these speculations, as are some heart disease drugs and anticancer drugs. While this is just speculation, it is better to err on the side of safety. If you are taking carbamazepine, citalopram, cyclosporine, clomimpramine, clozapine, fluoxetine, fluvoxamine, imipramine, naratriptan, olanzapine, paroxetine, phenobarbital, phenytoin, rizatriptan, sertraline, sumatriptan, theophylline, warfarin, or zolmitriptan, discuss your options with your healthcare professional. In some cases, close monitoring is in order; in some cases, temporarily discontinuing St. John's Wort makes the most sense, and in some cases, not taking St. John's Wort is most prudent.

The culprit seems to be hypericin, as it resembles substances that are known to induce enzymes that metabolize drugs. The following are facts:

> ➢ Studies are showing St. John's Wort preparations with varying amounts of hypericin don't seem to make a difference in the product's effectiveness as an antidepressant.

> ➢ Hypericin is likely an activator of the CYP450 enzyme system, which breaks down many drugs.

> ➤ Hypericin has been shown to not be the active ingredient in St. John's Wort.

Perhaps the time has come to remove hypericin and its related compounds from St. John's Wort and be done with it. Maybe it's time a "hypericin-free" St. John's Wort appeared on vitamin store shelves.

References:

See General Resources

Barbagallo, C. et al. "Antimicrobial Activity of Three Hypericum Species." *Filoterapia*. 1987; 58:175-77

Bennet, D, et al. "Neuropharmacology of St. John's Wort." *The Annals of Pharmacotherapy*. 1998' 5:245-252

Chatterjee, S, et al. "Hyperforin as a Possible Antidepressant Component of Hypericum Extracts." *Life Sci*. 1998; 63:499-510

DeSmet, P, et al. "St. John's Wort as an Antidepressant." *British Medical Journal*. 1996; 313:241-242

Ernst E. "St. John's Wort, An Anti-Depressant? A Systematic, Criteria Based Review." *Phytomed*. 1995; 2:67-71

Grube, B, et al. "St John's Wort extract: Efficacy for Menopausal Symptoms of Physiological Origin." *Adv Ther*. 1999; 16:177-186

Harrer, G, et al. "Treatment of Mild/Moderate Depressions with Hypericum." *Phytomed*. 1994; 1:3-8

Harrer, G, et al. "Comparison of Equivalence Between the St. John's Wort Extract LoHyp-57 and fluoxetine." *Arzneim-Forch Drug Res*. 1999; 49:289-96

Hobbs, C. "St. John's Wort: A Review." *HerbalGram*. 1989; 18/19: 24-33

Holzl, J. "Constituents and Mechanism of Action of St. John's Wort." *Zeitschr Phytother*. 1993; 14:255-64

Johne, A, et al. "Pharmacokinetic Interaction of Digoxin with an Herbal Extract from St. John's Wort." *Clin Pharmacol Ther*. 1999; 66:338-345

Laakmann, G. et al. "St. John's Wort in Mild to Moderate Depression: The Prevalence of Hyperforin for the Clinical Efficacy." *Pharmcopsychiatry*. 1998; 31:54-9

Lenoir, S, et al. "A Double-Blind Randomized Trial to Investigate Three Different Concentrations of a Standardized Fresh Plant Extract Obtained from the Shoots Tips of Hypericum Perforatum." *Phytomedicine.* 1999; 6:141-146

Martinez, B, et al. "Hypericum in the Treatment of Seasonal Affective Disorders." *J Ger Psychiatry Neural.* 1994; 1:S29-S33

Muller, W, et al. "Effects of Hypericum Extract (LI 160) in Biochemical Models of Antidepressant Activity." *Pharmacopsychiatry.* 1997; 30:102-7

Murray, M. "Common Questions About St. John's Wort Extract." *American Journal of Natural Medicine.* 1997; 4:14-19

O'Hara, M, et al. "A Review of 12 Commonly Used Medicinal Herbs." *Arch Fam Med.* 1998; 7:523-536

Philipp, M, et al. "Hypericum Extract versus Imipramine or Placebo in Patients with Moderate Depression: Randomized Multicenter Study of Treatment for Eight Weeks." *BMJ.* 1999; 319:1534-1538

Schultz, v, et al. *Rational Phytotherapy: A Physicians' Guide to Herbal Medicine.* Berlin. Springer. 1998

Schrader, E. "Equivalence of St. John's Wort Extract (Ze 117) and Fluoxetine: A Randomized, Controlled Study in Mild-Moderate Depression." *Int Clin Psychopharmacol.* 2000; 15:61-8

Stevinson, C, et al. "Hypericum for Fatigue- A Pilot Study." *Phytomedicine.* 1998; 5:443-447

Vorbach, E, et al. "Effectiveness and Tolerance of the Hypericum Extract LI 160 in Comparison with Imipramine: Randomized Double-Blind Study with 135 Patients." *J Ger Psychiatry Neurol.* 1994; 7:S19-S23

Wheatley, D. "Hypericum in Seasonal Affective Disorder." *Cur Med Res Opin.* 1999; 15:33-7

Uva Ursi

(Arctostaphylos uva-ursi)

Other Common Names:

Bearberry, Upland Cranberry, Mountain Cranberry, Wild Cranberry, Arberry, Hog Berry, Ptarmigan Berry, Redberry, Rockberry, Sandberry, Mealberry, Fox Berry, Universe Vine, Mountain Box, Bear's Grape, Kinnikinnick, Sagackhomi, Barren Myrtle

Background:

With at least twelve common names referring to a berry, what part of this plant do you think is used for medicine? Let me give you a hint. Uva Ursi means Bearberry in Latin, and Arctostaphylos means Bearberry in Greek. The answer is…the dried leaves are the only part used. Oh well.

Uva Ursi is a small evergreen shrub, similar to California's Manzanita, and native to the Northern Hemisphere. It grows wild in the north of America, Europe, and Asia, with medicinal material coming mostly from Italy, Spain and the Balkans. Native Americans used it for inflammation of the urinary tract.

Uva Ursi was used by the Greek healer, Galen (130-200 AD), as an astringent to stop bleeding. However, the plant was first properly documented in a Welsh herbal in the 13th century. And, it wasn't until the late 18th century that Spanish and Italian physicians began using it as a diuretic and astringent for diseases of the bladder and kidneys. In 1788, it was listed in the *London Pharmacopoeia*. In 1820, it became an official drug of the *United States Pharmacopoeia and National Formulary*, which lasted until 1950.

We're not sure whether Uva Ursi gets its name, Bearberry or Bear's Grape, because bear relish its taste or because the berry tastes so bad, only a bear could eat it.

Science:

Uva Ursi's leaves contain a phenolic glycoside called Arbutin, which ranges in concentration from 5% to 15%. In the presence of gastric fluid, Arbutin is metabolized to hydoquinone, which possess antiseptic and astringent properties. There is also evidence that Arbutin has antiseptic activity in its own right since it has been shown to have antimicrobial effects outside the body.

Other plant fractions, namely the triterpene derivative, Ursolic Acid, and the flavonoid, Isoquercitrin, are responsible for Uva Ursi's diuretic effect. The Allantoin content is known for its soothing and tissue rebuilding properties.

Modern Day Uses:

Uva Ursi is prescribed by herbalists for disorders of the bladder and kidneys, particularly in the presence of inflammation. It is a diuretic, soothing tonic, antiseptic, and disinfectant. It is also a good solvent for urinary calculi deposits.

Consider Uva Ursi for:

> - Urinary tract infections
> - Inflammation of the urinary tract
> - Cystitis
> - Urethritis
> - Water retention
> - Dysuria
> - Kidney stones
> - Urinary tonic

Dose:

Clinical grade Uva Ursi is generally standardized to 20-25% Arbutin. The dosage is calculated as 100-200 mg Arbutin 3-4 times daily.

Uva Ursi is a better antiseptic if it is working in alkaline urine. Therefore, if one were looking for its anti-infective benefits, it would be better to temporarily adjust one's diet to avoid acid forming foods. Avoid animal protein, and eat more vegetables. Another alternative is to artificially alkalize the urine by ingesting some bicarbonate of soda.

Cautions:

Excessive amounts of Uva Ursi may cause some stomach distress. Keep this in mind if you are starting off with a distressed stomach.

Uva Ursi may turn the urine a shade of greenish brown. Don't panic, this is harmless.

References:

See General Resources

DerMarderosian, A ed. *Review of Natural Products*. St. Louis, MO, Facts and Comparisons, 1999

Lloyd, J, et al. *Kings American Dispensatory*. 18th ed. Portland, OR, Eclectic Medical Publications. 1983

Uvae Ursi Folium. ESCOP Monograph, 1997

Valerian

(Valeriana officinalis)

Other Common Names:

Baldrian, Radix Valerianae, Indian Valerian, Red Valerian, All Heal, Great Wild Valerian

Background:

Secret of the Pied Piper

The first century Greek physician, Dioscorides, called Valerian, *Phu*, which is what he exclaimed when he smelled his roommate's jogging shoes, and likened it to Valerian's wonderful aroma. This disagreeable odor comes from the volatile oils in Valerian, and it is supposed to be attractive to rats. Legend has it that it was Valerian that the Pied Piper of Hamelin used to lead the little critters from his village.

I'm not sure about the rat legend, but cats are attracted to Valerian's smell, which is reminiscent of Catnip. Actually, in the 1700s, pharmacists determined the quality of their Valerian by how cats reacted to it. I was thinking of using my cat, Ginseng, to test my jogging shoes. When she gets out of control, it is time to buy a new pair.

A late bloomer as a nerve tonic

Galen, the last of the great Greek physicians, prescribed Valerian to induce sleep and to treat epilepsy. But, it wasn't until the Italian Fabio Colonna, who, in the late 1500s, cured himself of epilepsy, that Valerian became known primarily as a nervine and sedative. However, over the years, it has been used for a wide array of conditions including muscle spasms, as a sedative, for insomnia, nervous tension, fatigue, menstrual cramps, digestive problems, urinary tract disorders, flatulence, nausea, colic diarrhea, nervous heart conditions, anorexia in children, and inner unrest.

The genus Valeriana contains about 250 different species spread over the temperate regions of North America, Europe, South Africa, and southeastern South America. However, it is Valeriana officinalis that is commonly used as medicine around the world. V. officinalis is native to Europe but is now commonly seen growing wild along the roads of New England and adjacent areas. Its name is derived from the Latin *valeo*, which translates to "being strong" or *valere*, "being in health."

Valerian was an official remedy in the *U.S. Pharmacopoeia* from 1820 to 1936, and it is still an official drug listed in the pharmacopoeias of Austria, Britain, Czechoslovakia, Egypt, Europe, France, Germany, Greece, Hungary, Italy, Netherlands, Norway, Romania, Russia, Switzerland, and Yugoslavia. In the past few decades, hundreds of clinical studies have been reported and have validated Valerian as a mild sedative, mild analgesic, spasm reliever, and treatment for insomnia and nervous excitability.

Science:
The sedating actives in Valerian lay in the volatile oil of the roots, which contain three distinct classes of compounds. The first are its mono and sesquiterpenes, highlighted by valerenic acid. The second are its iridoid triesters, best exemplified by its valepotriates. The last class is its pyridine alkaloids, which take on a lesser role. These compounds are found exclusively in Valerian.

Oops
We used to think that only the valepotriates were responsible for Valerian's sedative effect, and medicines were standardized to them. However, when aqueous extracts were found to be effective relaxants, it was concluded that valerenic acid was also active because valepotriates are not soluble in water. Because of the instability of valepotriates and question of their safety, Valerian preparations are now generally standardized to valerenic acid or total volatile oil.

The root can contain between .4 and 1.5% volatile oil. Since concentration and composition of Valerian's volatile oil varies so greatly, standardization is highly desirable. Most monographs on Valerian require a minimum of .5% volatile oil. Other medicinal preparations are standardized to .8% valerenic acid.

How it works

The mechanism of action for the active constituents was only eluci-dated in 1989, when Holzl and Godau discovered that Valerian worked by binding to benzodiazepine receptors. Several years later, Italian researchers demonstrated that Valerian's central nervous system activ-ity involved GABA receptor sites, GABA being a calming neurotrans-mitter.

Modern Day Uses:

Based on sound medicine, Valerian's sedative characteristics are unequivocal. This natural sedating effect makes it a valuable alterna-tive to support the treatment of the following:

> ➢ Insomnia (reduce latency to sleep, improve sleep quality, reduce night awakenings, increase dream recalls)
> ➢ Anxiety
> ➢ Stress
> ➢ Withdrawal from sedative drugs
> ➢ Agitation
> ➢ Restlessness
> ➢ Muscle cramps
> ➢ Intestinal spasms
> ➢ Hypertension (best in combination with other natural agents)

Valerian is non-addictive and does not cause the morning-after hang-over that most pharmaceutical hypnotic drugs cause. It achieves this benefit on the basis that it forms only weak bonds to receptor sites, unlike its synthetic drug counterparts.

Just because Valerian and Valium® are spelled similarly, doesn't mean that Valium® is made from Valerian. It is not. Nor are the two entities in any way related. They are very different. One is a potent synthetic drug, and the other is a mild plant medicine.

Dose:

Use a preparation standardized to .8%-1% valerenic acid, and take 150 mg to 300 mg, 30 to 60 minutes before bedtime. Keep in mind that, as a nervous system tonic, Valerian may take up to four weeks to improve mood and sleep disorders.

Valerian is very non-toxic. An intentional overdose has been reported in which 20 times the recommended dose was slugged down. Everybody lived happily ever after, following 24 hours of mild symptoms. The moral of this story is that if you want to do yourself in, pick something else to do it with, and, if you need to take a little over the normal dose to get to sleep under dire straits, don't worry about it.

For daytime anxiety use, I like combination preparations using smaller doses of Valerian coupled with other calming agents like, oats, passion flower, lemon balm, skullcap, kava, etc.

Cautions:

There has been some concern raised over the possibility that valepotriates might have mutagenic properties, based on their alkylating and cytotoxic activity in cell cultures. I believe that this is much to do about nothing. First of all, valepotriates are highly unstable and extremely poorly absorbed in the body, making them a dubious source of toxicity. Secondly, clinical investigators concluded that intracellular nucleophiles bind and neutralize them, protecting the cell against any cytotoxic effect. So there!

Although Valerian will generally not interfere with motor functions, if you take enough Valerian for sleep, don't sleep and drive, or operate machinery. And since not drinking and driving is already a rule, don't drink, take Valerian, and drive. And last, but not least, it is not a good idea to take Valerian and other depressant or hypnotic drugs. They can have an additive effect.

Valerian has been used during pregnancy and lactation, and European laboratory studies have shown no harmful effects, but don't try this at home. Discuss using any botanical with your herb-savvy health care professional.

References:

See General Resources

Bos, R. et al. "Cytotoxic Potential of Valerian Constituents and Valerian Tinctures." *Phytomedicine*. 1998; 5:219-225

Brown, D. "Valerian: Clinical Overview." *Townsend Letter for Doctors*. 1995; 150-51

Holzl, J. & Godau, P. "Receptor Bindings Studies with Valeriana officinalis on the Benzodiazepine Receptor." *Planta Medica*. 1989; 55;642

Kuhlmann, J, et al. "The Influence of Valerian Treatment on 'Reaction Time,' Alertness and Concentration." *Pharmacopsychiat*. 1999; 32:235-41

Leathwood, P. et al. "Aqueous Extract of Valerian Root Improves Sleep Quality in Man." *Pharmacology, Biochemistry & Behavior*. 1982; 17:65-71

Leathwood, P. et al. "Aqueous Extract of Valerian Reduces Latency to Fall Asleep in Man." *Planta Med*. 1985; 51:144-8

Leuschner, J. et al. "Characterization of the Central Nervous Depressant Activity of Commercially Available Valerian Root Extract." *Arzneimittelforschung*. 1993; 43:638-41

Lindahl, G, et al. "Double-Blind Study of a Valerian Preparation." *Pharmacol Biochem Behav*. 1989; 32:1065-6

Mennini, T, et al. "*In Vitro* Study on the Interaction of Extracts and Pure Compounds from Valeriana Officinalis Roots with GABA, Benzodiazepine and Barbiturate Receptors." *Fitoterapia*. 1993; 64:291-300

O'Hara, M, et al. "A Review of 12 Commonly Used Medicinal Herbs." *Arch Fam Med*. 1998; 7:523-536

White Willow Bark

(Salix alba)

Other Common Names:
Willow, Weidenrinde

Background:
The Willow is a shrub or tree depending on its size (some can grow to 50 feet), native to England, Europe, Asia, and North America. There are 300 species of Salix we call Willow, White Willow being just one of them. Some of Willow's applications come to us from the Greeks, Dioscorides reporting therapeutic uses for gout and rheumatic joint diseases in his herbal *De Materia Medica* (1st century AD). Ancient Egyptians used the bark, as we do today, for pain and inflammation. And, closer to home, our Native Americans relied on Willow for its analgesic properties.

In 1829, another bright pharmacist, this time a Frenchman named H. Leroux, discovered Willow's active chemical, salicin. In 1838, pure salicylic acid was synthesized by an Italian chemist, not from Willow but Wintergreen and other plants. Salicin and salicylic acid were widely used through the 19th century for fever, gout, pain, and inflammation. However, as usual, when you isolate chemicals from plants or synthesize them, you almost always increase their toxicity. The farther away you stray from Nature, the more likely you are to do harm. And such was the case. The high doses used routinely led to gastric irritation and vomiting. Based on autopsy reports, there may have even been a relationship between Ludwig Von Beethoven's renal disease and the use of powdered salicylates.

Then came the discovery of the millennium. In 1893, Felix Hoffman at the Bayer Company in Germany, following French studies of 1853, was able to synthesize acetylsalicylic acid from a chemical called "spirin" found in Meadowsweet. And so, Bayer Aspirin® was born. And things haven't been the same since. Not only did aspirin do everything that its natural counterparts did, today it is even used to

prevent heart attacks, strokes, and colorectal cancer. Bayer Aspirin®
has become one of the most popular drugs sold in the world.

Since the development of aspirin in the 1890s, White Willow has fallen
into disuse. However, don't count it out. It may still have some
benefits over its synthetic counterpart.

Science:

White Willow phytochemically consists of glycosides (.5-11%),
tannins, aromatic aldehydes and acids, and flavonoids. Its actives are
its salicylate-forming glycosides, namely salicin and salicortin. Salicin
and salicortin are metabolized by intestinal flora to something called
saligenin, which is absorbed into the bloodstream and is metabolized
by the liver to salicylic acid. This is the active compound that is
eventually excreted by the kidney.

The mechanism by which salicylic acid works is the same as aspirin.
That is, it inhibits cyclooxygenase enzymes, which are involved in
prostaglandin synthesis.

So, what are the benefits of nature over synthetics?

➤ White Willow does not interfere with coagulation. It does
not prolong bleeding times, nor does it inhibit platelet
aggregation. Aspirin is the only salicylate to contain an
acetyl group. This acetyl group is transferred and irrevers-
ibly bound to cyclooxygenase-1 in platelets, therefore
inhibiting aggregation. No acetyl group…no thrombolytic
effect.

➤ White Willow actives are considered pro-drugs. That is,
they are converted by the liver into their active salicylic
acid state. This by-passes the gastrointestinal tract, thereby
avoiding GI irritation.

➤ According to the German Federal Institute of Pharmaceutical and Medicinal Products, there is no evidence that
Willow preparations should be contraindicated in small
children with flu for fear of producing Reyes syndrome; the

salicylates in Willow metabolize differently than aspirin (acetylsalicylic acid).

➤ While Willow has a slower onset of action and a longer duration of action, thereby allowing for a longer dosing interval.

Modern Day Uses:
White Willow can be used for:

➤ Arthritic and rheumatoid pain
➤ Backaches
➤ Low back pain
➤ Gout
➤ Neuralgia
➤ Muscle pain
➤ Any chronic pain
➤ Fever
➤ Headaches
➤ Symptoms of colds and flu

Dose:
Dosing is generally 60-120 mg (total salicin) daily, not to exceed 240 mg.

For chronic pain, lessening is usually seen in the first few days, but best results come in the next one to four weeks of use.

To obtain more potency, look for preparations that combine salicylic acid pro-phytochemicals from different herbs. Examples are: Purple Willow, Meadowsweet, Aspen, and Wintergreen

Cautions:
None known.

References:

See General Resources

Hedner, T, et al. "The Early Clinical History of Salicylates in Rheumatology and Pain." *Clinical Rheumatology*. 1998; 17:17-25

Fotsch, G, et al. "Biotransformation of Phenol Glycosides Leiocarposide and Salicin." *Phamrazie*. 1989; 44:555-8

Julkunen-Titto, R, et al. "The Enzymatic Decomposition of Salicin and Its Derivatives Obtained from Salicacae Species." *J Ntl Prod*. 1992; 55:1204-12

Meier, B, et al. "Identification and Determination of 8 Phenol Glycosides Each in Salix Purpurea and S. Daphnoides by Modern HPLC." *Pharmaceutica Acta Helvetiae*. 1985; 60:269-75

Robbers, J, Tyler, V, et al. *Pharmacognosy and Pharmacobiotechnology*. Baltimore. Williams & Wilkins. 1996

Schwartz, A. "Beethoven's Renal Disease Based on His Autopsy: A Case of Papillary Necrosis." *Am J Kidney Dis*. 1993; 21:643-52

Vainio, H, et al. "Aspirin for The Second Hundred Years: New Uses for an Old Drug." *Pharmacology & Toxicology*. 1997; 81:151-2

Weiss, H, et al. " The Effects of Salicylates on the Hemostatic Properties of Platelets in Man." *J Clin Inv*. 1968; 47:2169-80

Yarrow

(Achillea millefolium)

Other Common Names:

Thousand-Leaf, Thousand Weed, Milfoil, Knight's Milfoil, Green Arrow, Wound Wort, Soldier's Wound Wort, Nosebleed Plant, Bloodwort, Gordaldo, Old Man's Pepper, Sanguinary, Stanchgrass, Thousand Seal, Dog Daisy, Ladies' Mantle, Noble Yarrow, Devil's Nettle, Devil's Plaything, Bad Man's Plaything, Yarroway, Carpenter's Weed

Background:

Yarrow is an ancient herb that originated in Europe, and is now naturalized in temperate regions throughout the world. Since medieval times it has been much esteemed as a wound herb, as some of its common names imply (Knight's Milfoil, Soldier's Wound Wort). It was called *Herba Militaris*, which further suggests its use for battle wounds.

The English botanist, John Gerard (1545-1612), wrote that Yarrow is the same plant with which Achilles treated the bleeding of his soldiers, hence the genus name *Achillea*. According to the Anglo-Saxon version of the *Herbarium Apuleii Platoni* (11th century) notes: "It is said that Achilles the chieftain found it, and he with this same wort healed them who were stricken and wounded with iron." The mythological legend is that Telephus, son of Hercules, wounded by Achilles' spear, was told by an oracle, that his wounder would be his healer. Achilles agreed to help, in return for assistance in getting to Troy. He scraped some rust from his spear from which sprang the plant Yarrow and this healed the wound.

The stalks of the plant, stripped of their leaves, were used to obtain hexagrams from the I Ching, the ancient Taoist Book of Oracles. The stalks are tossed to predict the future. Forty-nine sticks are divided into two piles and each of these piles are divided into fours. The remaining stalks add to form a line of the hexagram. I am not sure how this prophesizes the future, but I do know that this is the prototype of a I played as a child called "pick-up-sticks."

When you've been around as long as Yarrow, you can't help but have a colorful past. It has been used as a sneezing powder and for snuff. Chewing fresh leaves has been suggested to relieve toothaches. Dr. James Parkinson (1755-1824), for whom the disease is named, wrote that, "If it be put into the nose, assuredly it will stay the bleeding of it." And, it was brought to weddings to ensure seven years love (after that you were on your own). Yarrow was an official drug, listed in the United States Pharmacopoeia from 1863-82, used as a tonic, stimulant and emmenagogue (an agent that induces or increases menstrual flow.)

A useful plant in the garden, Yarrow attracts butterflies as well as ladybugs and parasitic wasps that prey on aphids. Yarrow added to the compost pile will speed decomposition.

Science:
There are about 85 species of Yarrow, from which 123 constituents of know pharmacological activity have been identified. The following represents an abbreviated list:

> ➤ Volatile oil- from which 82 constituents have been documented including, azulenes, eugenol, caryphyllene, jumulene, limonene, sabinene, thujone, borneol and camphor.
> ➤ Flavonoids- including, luteolin, apigenin, kaempferol and quercitrin.
> ➤ Bitters- including the sesquiterpenes
> ➤ Alkaloids- including achilleine, stachydrine
> ➤ Coumarins, resin, , asparagin, tannins, aconitic and isovalerianic acids, sterols

Because of the commonalties between yarrow species, it has been assumed by some that "Yarrow is Yarrow." The reality is that some varieties contain no chamazulene, the phytochemical that goes to anti-inflammatory activity. The only species that contains thujone, a substance that Yarrow's presumed efficacy in treating menstrual problems, is true Yarrow, *Achillea millefolium*. And, there are probably other important differences between chemical profiles that are not even know yet.

Some constituents of the plant have been shown to be peripheral vasodilators, particularly on venous circulation that may help improve circulation, help hemorrhoids, tone varicose veins, and lower high blood pressure.

Yarrow is diaphoretic and antipyretic, meaning it induces perspiraton and lowers fever. It was once a popular substitute for quinine. It is a bitter, making it a digestive tonic, carminative and antispasmodic. It is a styptic (stops bleeding) and antiseptic, making it a wound healer. And, as a women's herb, it is a menstrual regulator, emmenagogue, and restrains excessive menstrual bleeding.

Modern Day Uses:

Taken as a hot tea, Yarrow is excellent for inducing perspiration and lowering fever of colds and flu. Women may consider it, or identify it in combination remedies for various female health irregularities or disorders. Yarrow can be used as a digestive tonic. And, you may find it included in herbal combination remedies for varicose veins and hemorrhoids among many of the above mentions ailments.

If you find no other use for Yarrow, try this. Put an ounce of the herb sewed up in flannel and place it under your pillow. Repeat the words:

> *Thou pretty herb of Venus's tree,Thy true name it is Yarrow;Now who my bosom friend must be,Pray tell me thou me tomorrow.*

This will bring forth a vision of your future love.

Dose:

Yarrow can be administered as a tea or powdered in capsules. Follow label instructions.

Cautions:

The relative short duration of use, or, the fact that Yarrow will often be included as part of a combination formula, nullify any toxicity or interactions that may be speculated. Yarrow is considered to be non-toxic. Some research indicates that mild skin rashes can occur in allergic people.

References:

See General Resources

DerMarderosian, A ed. *Review of Natural Products*. St. Louis, MO, Facts and Comparisons, 1999

Grieve, M. *A Modern Herbal*. New York, NY. Dover Publications. 1971

Mabey, R. *the New Age Herbalist*. New York, NY. Simon & Schuster. 1988Van Hevelinger, A. "Fair Yarrows."*The Herb Companion*. 1996; 47-53

Zeylstra, H. "Just Yarrow?" *British Journal of Phytotherapy*. 1997; 4:184-89

Yucca

(Yucca spp.)

Other Common Names:
Dagger Plant, Soapweed, Our-Lord's Candle, Adam' Needle, Bear Grass, Spanish Bayonet, Joshua Tree

Background:
As many as 40 species of trees and shrubs found mostly in the deserts of North America are referred to as Yucca. The Yucca species, in addition to other agaves and tequila starting materials, have in common that they contain large amounts of saponins. These are bitter substances that foam when shaken with water—like soap. In fact, Native Americans used them in soap, in addition to using the fiber for rope, sandals, and clothing.

Another thing that Yucca plants have in common is that they depend on a nocturnal yucca moth, called Tegeticula. The Tegeticula genus contains four species that have adapted to a species of Yucca. The moths emerge when the Yucca flowers open. The female gathers pollen from one flower, rolls it into a ball, flies to another flower, and lays eggs. The yucca can be fertilized by no other insect, and the moth can utilize no other plant. Marriage should work so well.

Yucca was used traditionally by Native Americans. The Cherokee used it to treat diabetes, for sores, and to reduce fevers. More modern Western herbalists have used, and continue to use it for arthritis, high blood pressure and digestive disorders. More widespread use of Yucca has been thwarted by its actives being elusive and requiring further research.

Science:
The roots of Yucca contain saponins that are steroid derivatives. Most species contain sarsasapogenin and tigogenin, the latter of which can be used as a starting point in the commercial synthesis of steroidal hormones.

Anti-inflammatory activity is observed in animal models. And, while not one of the best controlled studies ever done, one report concluded that giving Yucca for arthritis over a period of 15 months proved to be effective and safe. Interestingly enough, patients who received the Yucca for at least six months were found to have lower blood pressure, lower cholesterol, and lower incidence of migraine headaches. This would validate many of the traditional uses of Yucca.

Since saponins aren't absorbed orally that well, researchers are looking at other components of the plant. They have found two polysaccharides in an extract of the flowers of Y. glauca that have melanoma antitumor activity in mice. In addition, Yucca leaf protein has been found to inhibit certain viruses including Herpes.

Modern Day Uses:
Yucca may be beneficial for treating arthritis, migraine headaches, hyperlipidemia, and hypertension.

And if for nothing else, a panel of professional veterinary sniffers determined that, when added to cat and dog food, Yucca greatly reduced fecal odor. How does one end up with a job like that?

Dose:
Take a basic 4:1 extract, 500 mg 3-4 times daily.

Cautions:
None known.

References:
See General Resources

Ali, M, et al. "Isolation of Antitumor Polysaccharide Fractions from Yucca Glauca." *Growth.* 1978; 42:213

Bingham, R, et al. "Yucca Plant Saponin in Management of Arthritis." *J App Nut.* 1975; 27:45-51

Bull, J, et al. "Distinguishing Mechanisms for the Evolution of Cooperation." *J Theor Biol.* 1991; 149:63

Dewidar, A, et al. "The Steroid Sapogenin Constituents of Agave Americana, A. Variegata, and Y Gloriosa." *Plant Med.* 1970; 19:87

Hayashi, K, et al. "Yucca leaf Protein Sops the Protein Synthesis in HSV-Infected Cells and Inhibits Virus Replication." *Antiviral Res.* 1992; 17:323

Lowe, J, et al. *Research in Veterinary Science.* 1997; 63:61-66

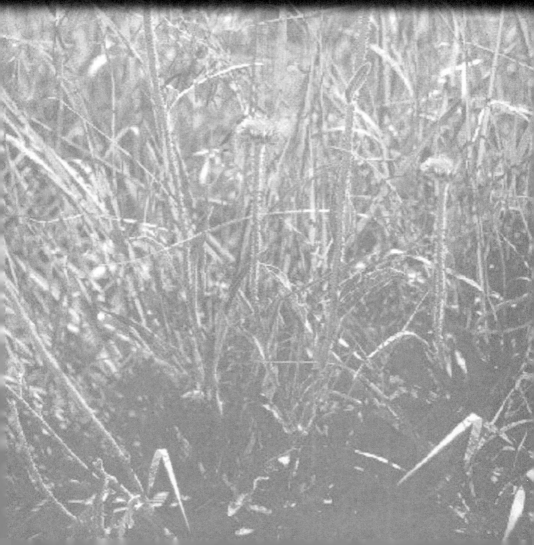

Part Three

Glossary

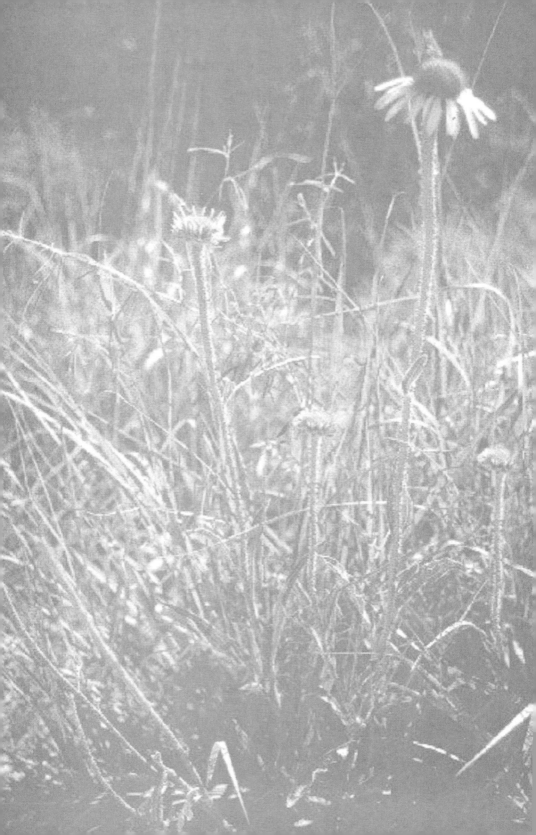

Glossary

Abortifacient- (noun), induces abortion

Abscess- (noun), encapsulated collection of pus and liquefied tissue

Acid- (adjective), having a pH less than 7 (neutral); opposite of alkaline

Acrid- (adjective), caustic, unpleasantly pungent, having a burning sensation in the mouth

Acute- (adjective), descriptive of a disorder with fast onset, short duration, and intense symptoms

Adaptogen – (noun), a botanical agent that strengthens organs or the entire body, increases resistance to stress and disease, tones and balances body systems

Adenitis- (Noun) inflammation of a gland or lymph nodes

Adhesion- (noun) a fibrous band holding parts of connective tissue together that are normally separated

Adipose- (adjective) fatty or pertaining to fat

Adjuvant- (adjective) that which assists or has an additive effect on another treatment

AIDS- (noun), acquired immune deficiency syndrome, severe weakening and subsequent destruction of immune system

Aldosterone- (noun), adrenal hormone that causes water retention

Alkaline- (adjective), having a pH above 7 (neutral), the opposite of acid

Alkaloid- (noun), a nitrogen-containing compound made by plants that reacts with acids to forms soluble salts that exert pronounced effects on bodily functions

Alterative- (noun), a plant that increases vitality through improving the breakdown and excretion of waste and toxins

Amino acid- (noun) nitrogen-containing compounds that are the building blocks of proteins

Anabolic- (adjective), promotes growth

Analgesic- (used as both a noun and an adjective), pain killer

Androgen- (noun), male hormones

Anemia- (noun), a condition in which hemoglobin content in the blood is less than that required to provide the oxygen demands of the body, results in fatigue

Angina- (noun), a crushing chest pain with a feeling of suffocation

Anodyne- (noun), a substance that relieves pain, synonym for analgesic.

Anorexia- (noun), lack of appetite, frequently seen in depression, commencement of fevers and illnesses

Anoxia- (noun), inadequate oxygen in body tissue

Anthelmintic- (noun), an agent that destroys parasitic intestinal worms

Anthocyanidin- (noun), a type of flavonoid typically showing as a pigment in the blue to red range

Anthraquinones- (noun0, glycoside compounds that produce dyes and purgatives

Antibacterial- (adjective), destroys or inhibits the growth of bacteria

Antibody- (noun), a protein made by the immune system in response to and interacting specifically with an antigen, by binding to and neutralizing it

Anticatarrhal- (used as both an adjective and a noun), relieving nasal congestion

Anticoagulant- (used as both an adjective and a noun), slows blood clotting

Antidote- (noun), poison neutralizer

Antigen- (noun), a substance perceived by the body as an invader that stimulates the immune system to respond by making an antibody against it

Antihypertensive- (used as both an adjective and a noun), a substance that lowers blood pressure

Antioxidant- (used as both adjective and noun), neutralizes free radicals

Antipeptic- (adjective), controls overproduction of digestive juices and enzymes

Antiperiodic- (adjective), prevents the reoccurrence of a disease that tends to come back

Antiphlogistic- (adjective), counteracts inflammation

Antipruritic- (adjective), relieves itching

Antiputrescent- (adjective), prevents decay

Antipyretic- (adjective), reduces fever

Antirheumatic- (adjective), quells symptoms of rheumatism

Antiseptic- (adjective), prevents infection by inhibiting the growth of infectious agents

Antispasmodic- (adjective), reduces contraction of muscle, usually involuntary muscle, quells spasms

Antitussive- (adjective), suppresses coughing

Anxiety- (noun), an emotional state ranging from mild unease to intense fear

Aphrodisiac- (adjective), stimulates sex drive

Apnea- (noun), a brief interruption of breathing

Apoplexy- (noun), sudden loss of consciousness followed by paralysis caused by hemorrhage into the brain, a stroke; formation of an embolus or thrombus that occludes an artery

Aprient- (noun), mild laxative

Arrhythmia- (noun), irregular heartbeat

Arteriosclerosis- (noun), hardening of the arteries

Aseptic- (adjective), free of disease-causing microorganisms

Astringent- (adjective), causing contraction of tissue by precipitating protein from the surface of cells; can reduce bleeding and discharges

Asymptomatic- (adjective) having an absence of symptoms of disease

Ataxia- (noun), unsteady gait; shaky movements

Atheroma- (noun), a fatty degeneration of artery walls due to plaque infiltration

Atherosclerosis- (noun), a disease process by which fats accumulate on inside of arteries

Atony- (noun), lack of muscle tone

Atrophy- (noun), wasting of organ due to cellular degeneration

Autoimmune- (adjective), descriptive of a disorder of defense mechanisms whereby antibodies are produced against body's own tissue

Autonomic nervous system- (noun), the part of the central nervous system responsible for control of bodily functions that are not consciously directed

Ayurvedic- (adjective), pertaining to Ayurveda, the Traditional Indian system of medicine

Bacteremia- (noun), bacteria in blood indicating infection

Bactericidal-(adjective), synonym—bacteriocidal, causing death of bacteria

Bile- (noun), a thick black fluid made by the liver and stored in the gallbladder that helps digest fats

Bitters- (noun), herbs with a bitter taste that stimulate the secretion of digestive juices and increase the functional tone of the gastrointestinal system

Blood sugar level- (noun), the concentration of glucose in the blood

Boil- (noun, a tender, inflamed, puss-filled area under the skin; a furuncle

Bronchial- (adjective), relating to the air passages

Bursitis- (noun), inflammation of the bursa, which is a pouch filled with lubricating fluid in a joint

Calculi- (noun), stones, actually pebble-like masses, called kidney stones when found in the kidney and gallstones when found in the gall bladder

Calmative- (adjective), sedative

Candidiasis- (noun), a yeast/fungus infection

Carbohydrate- (noun), sugars and starches

Carbuncle- (noun), a boil with multiple drainage channels

Carcinogen- (noun), a cancer-causing agent

Cardiotonic- (noun), tones and strengthens the heart

Carminative - (noun), prevents the formation or causes the expulsion of flatus, or put another way, an agent that relieves farting; relieves colic and digestive discomfort

Catarrh- (noun), excessive mucus in the membranes of the nose

Catecholamines- chemically similar neurotransmitters with marked effects on the nervous and cardiovascular systems, metabolic rate, temperature and smooth muscle including dopamine, epinephrine, and norepinephrine

Cathartic- (adjective), stimulating bowel movement

Caustic- (adjective), causing burning through chemical reaction

Cerebral- (adjective), pertaining to the largest part of brain, the cerebrum

Chemotypes- (noun), plants from the same species that, due to environmental differences, contain different chemical constituents but are otherwise botanically indistinguishable

Chilblains- (noun), swollen itchy red skin on fingers and toes due to cold

Cholagogue- (noun), a substance that stimulates gallbladder contraction and thus the release of bile

Cholecystitis- (noun), inflammation of the gallbladder

Cholelithiasis- (noun), gallstones

Choleretic- (adjective), promoting the flow of bile

Cholestasis- (noun), liver congestion

Cholinergic- (adjective), pertaining to the parasympathetic nervous system and its neurotransmitter, acetylcholine

Chromatography- (noun), a process that separates chemical compounds

Chronic fatigue syndrome- (noun), chronic weakness and extreme exhaustion due to unknown causes

Chronic- (adjective), long-term

Cirrhosis- (noun), liver disease characterized by cell scaring

Claudication- (noun), cramps and pain resulting from inadequate blood supply to muscle

CNS- (noun), central nervous system, the brain and spinal cord

Cold sore- (noun), a blister-like sore in or around the mouth, usually viral in origin

Colic- (noun), a spasmodic pain in any hollow or tubular organ, eg. the colon, that comes in waves

Colitis- (noun), inflammation of colon

Complement- (noun) a set of enzymes that work with antibodies to attack foreign invaders

Compress- (noun), a pad, soaked in a solution that is then held in place on the skin

Congestive Heart Failure- (noun), inability of the heart to supply the oxygen needs of the body

Connective tissue- (noun), tissue that supports and connects other tissues and parts, acting like cement to hold cells together

Constipation- (noun), infrequent, difficult, or painful bowel movements; hard stools; irregularity

Contagious- (adjective), spreading from person to person

Contraceptive- (noun), any process, device or method that prevents pregnancy

Contraindication- (noun), a preexisting condition or disease that would preclude the use of a substance because medical knowledge reveals that a certain substance will tend to produce an adverse reaction and exacerbate the pathology

Contusion- (noun), bruise

Cooling remedy- (noun), usually a bitter or relaxant herb that reduces internal body heat usually by clearing toxins

Corticosteriod hormones- (noun), adrenal gland hormones whose primary functions are inflammation, body fluid control, suppression of the immune response, controlling the body's use of nutrients

Cortisol- (noun), an adrenal stress hormone that regulates organic metabolism by converting fats and proteins to glucose

Cortisone- (noun), an adrenal hormone that counteracts pain and swelling

Coumarin- (noun), a vanilla-scented plant constituent that can aid in blood thinning

Counterirritant- (noun), a substance that causes superficial irritation of skin, increasing blood flow, speeding removal of toxins, and subsequently relieving inflammation of deeper tissue

Crohn's disease- (noun), a chronic inflammation and thickening of the lining of the gut

Cutaneous- (adjective) pertaining to the skin

Cyanosis- (noun), a bluish, grayish or dark purple discoloration of the skin due to the presence of abnormal amounts of reduced hemoglobin in the blood, or in other words, due to a lack of oxygenated blood

Cyst-(noun), a liquid filled lump

Cystitis- (noun), a bladder inflammation generally due to infection

Cytotoxic- (adjective), toxic to all cells

Cytotoxin- (noun), a substance that is toxic to certain cells, used against certain tumors

Debility- (noun), a weakness

Decoctions- (noun), teas prepared by cooking plant material in boiling water

Dehydration- (noun), water loss

Dementia- (noun), senility

Demulcent- (noun), a soothing agent

Depressant- (noun) a sedative

Depurative- (adjective), promoting elimination of waste

Dermatitis- (noun), skin inflammation

Detoxicant- (noun), a substance that removes poisons

Diaphoretic- (adjective), causing sweating, thus lowering fever

Digestive- (noun), herbs that promote or aid digestion

Disaccharide- (noun), a sugar composed of two single units

Disinfectant- (noun) a cleansing agent that destroys microbes

Diuretic- (used as a noun and adjective), causes urination

Diverticulitis- (noun), inflammation of sac-like pouches in the gut

Dopamine- (noun), a neurotransmitter, precursor to epinephrine and norepinephrine

Double-blind- (adjective), a type of study in which neither party knows who is getting the test substance

Dropsy- (noun), a condition in which excessive fluid builds up in the tissues

Dysentery- (noun), an intestinal infection characterized by severe diarrhea with blood

Dysfunction- (noun), a malfunction

Dysmenorrhea- (noun), painful or difficult menstruation

Dyspepsia- (noun), pain and gas after eating, sometimes with nausea, vomiting; indigestion

Dysplasia- (noun) abnormal cellular growth

Dyspnea- (noun), difficulty breathing

Edema- (noun), fluid accumulation

Embolism- (noun), an artery obstruction caused by a dislodged blood clot

Emetic- (adjective), causing vomiting

Emmenagogue- (noun), a substance that stimulates and normalizes menstrual flow

Emollient- (adjective), softens skin

Emulsify- (verb), to disperse large fat globules into smaller uniformly distributed particles

Endemic- (noun), a disease chronically present in a particular region or population but that has low mortality, such as measles

Endocrine gland- (noun), a ductless organ that releases hormones directly into the bloodstream

Endometriosis- (noun), an inflammation of endometrial tissue, frequently forming cysts containing altered blood

Endometrium- (noun), the mucus membrane lining of the uterus

Endorphin- (noun), a pain killing, feel good neurotransmitter

Enteritis- (noun), infectious inflammation of the small intestine

Enuresis- (noun), involuntary urination, bedwetting

Enzyme- (noun), a protein catalyst that bridges the completion of a reaction

Essential oils- (noun), a complex mixture of organic compounds that evaporate when exposed to air; usually the odiferous components of plants

Estrogenic- (adjective), similar in effects to estrogen

Estrogens- (noun), female hormones

Euphoric- (noun), a substance that causes an increased sense of well being

Excitant- (noun), a substance that causes stimulation

Excretion- (verb), waste elimination process by the body

Exfoliant- (noun), a substance that causes sloughing of unwanted tissue

Expectorant- (noun), a substance that thins mucus in the respiratory tract encouraging its elimination

Extract- (noun), the concentrated form of a natural substance; involves the use of solvents to dissolve solids so that they can be recovered as a concentrate.

Exudate- (noun), that which oozes from the body

Febrifuge- (noun), a substance that lowers fever

Fissure- (noun), a crack

Fistula- (noun), an abnormal tube-like passage from a normal cavity or tube to a free surface or to another cavity; may be due to congenital defect or result from abcesses, injuries or inflammatory processes

Flatus- (noun), fart

Flavonoid- (noun), a member of a chemical family that contains flavones, usually pigment chemicals whose job it is, in the plant, to protect against damaging substances

Free radical- (noun), highly reactive unstable molecules that, if not neutralized, can bind with and destroy cellular compounds

Fungicide- (noun), a substance that destroys fungus

Furuncle- (noun), a boil

Galactogogue-(noun), a substance that increases breast milk flow

Gallstone- (noun), a hard mass of bile, cholesterol, and calcium salts

Gastric ulcer- (noun), a stomach ulcer

Gastritis- (noun), an inflammation of the stomach lining

Gastroenteritis- (noun), an inflammation of the stomach and intestines

Genital herpes- (noun), a lesion on the genitals caused by the herpes simplex virus

Genitourinary- (adjective), relating to both reproductive and urinary systems

Genus- (noun), a plant category, below family and above species

Germicidal- (adjective), kills germs

Gingivitis- (noun), an inflammation of the gums

Glaucoma- (noun), an eye condition characterized by intraocular pressure

Glucose- (noun), the simplest form of sugar used by the body for fuel

Glycoprotein- (noun), a carbohydrate-protein complex

Glycoside- (noun), an active plant constituent that contains a sugar (glycone) and a non-sugar (aglycone) part; cardioactive, purgative

Glycosuria- (noun), excessive sugar in the urine

Gout- (noun), excessive uric acid in the blood, causing joint pain and kidney stones

Grippe- (noun), the flu

Gum- (noun), a class of carbohydrate that swells in water

HDL- (noun), high-density lipoprotein; the good guy that removes cholesterol from arteries

Hematoma- (noun), a bruise, typically with black and blue discoloration

Hematuria- (noun), blood in the urine

Hemostatic- (adjective), stops bleeding

Hepatic herb- (adjective + noun), an herb that aids liver function

Herbal- (noun), a comprehensive publication on herbs

Herpes- (noun), a virus causing small viral blisters on the skin

HIV- (noun), human immunodeficiency virus, causes AIDS

Hives- (noun), round, red itchy welts on skin

Hormone- (noun), a chemical substance produced by a gland that travels through the blood to a certain tissue, on which it exerts an effect

Hyperglycemia- (noun), high blood sugar

Hyperlipidemia- (noun), high blood fats: cholesterol, triglycerides

Hyperplasia- (noun), an increase in the number of cells in a tissue or organ

Hypertension- (noun), high blood pressure

Hypertensive herb- (noun), an herb that raises blood pressure

Hyperthermia- (noun), a fever of 105 degrees or higher

Hypertrophy-(noun), increase in size of tissue due to cellular enlargement

Hyperventilation- (noun), abnormally rapid breathing, with the effect of lowering carbon dioxide in the blood

Hypnotic- (adjective), induces sleep

Hypoglycemia- (noun), low blood sugar

Hypoglycemic herb- (noun), an herb that lowers blood sugar

Hypotensive herb- (noun), an herb that lowers blood pressure

Hypothermia- (noun), body temperature below normal

Hypoxia- (noun), low oxygen supply

Hysteria- (noun), a disorder characterized by emotional outbursts

Immune system- (noun), the complex of organs, cells, tissues and proteins that work in a coordinated manner to defend the body against invading pathogens such as viruses and bacteria

Immunostimulant herb- (noun), an herb that stimulates the immune system

Impairment- (noun), damage or weakening of a body junction or part

Impetigo- (noun), a contagious bacterial skin infection

In Vitro- (adverb), Latin for outside the body; usually in an artificial environment such as a test tube

In Vivo- (adverb), Latin for inside the body

Incontinence- (noun), inability to control urination; welcome to Depends®

Incubation period- (noun), the time between exposure to an infectious disease and the onset of its symptoms, during which an infection is developing

Infusion- (noun), a preparation made by steeping herbs in hot water; a tea

Insomnia- (noun), inability to sleep

Insulin- (noun), a sugar-lowering hormone secreted by pancreas

Interferon- (noun), viral and cancer killing substance made by the immune system

Irritable bowel syndrome- (noun), chronic pain with constipation and/or diarrhea caused by contractions of colon muscle; spastic colon

Ischemia- (noun), reduced blood supply to tissue

Jaundice- (noun), yellow skin due to elevation of bilirubin in the body; liver disease symptom

Kidney stone- (noun), a hard pebble-like mass in the kidney; a calculus

Lactation- (noun), the secretion of milk from the mammary glands

Laxative- (noun), a substance that promotes emptying of the bowels

LDL- (noun) low-density lipoprotein; the bad guy that delivers cholesterol to arteries

Lesion- (noun), a localized abnormal tissue formation

Lethargy- (noun), lack of energy

Leukotrienes- (noun), inflammatory compound

Lichen- (noun), a harmonic relationship between algae and fungus

Lignan- (noun), a plant material that binds cellulose fibers in wood

Lipase- (noun) a fat-degrading enzyme

Lipids- (noun), fat substances present in most tissues that are important structural materials in the body

Lubricant- (noun), a substance that reduces friction

Lumbago- (noun), lower back pain

Lumen- (noun), the area within a tube

Lupus- (noun), an autoimmune disease that causes skin complications, joint pain, and organ damage

Macerate- (verb), in herbal medicine, to soak a substance, typically in a solution of alcohol and water, until it is soft

Malabsorption- (noun), impaired absorption of nutrients

Malaise- (noun), a vague nondescript feeling of being sick

Malignant- (adjective), descriptive of a condition that worsens and usually causes death

Mastitis- (noun), inflammation of the breast, usually due to infection

Materia medica- (noun), a publication that is a comprehensive scientific study of medicinal substances, their sources, preparation, and use

Menorrhagia- (noun), excessive bleeding during menses

Menstruation- (noun), that part of the female cycle when the lining of the uterus is broken down and discharged as blood and debris

Metabolite- (noun), a product of a chemical reaction

Molecule-(noun), the smallest complete unit of a substance

Mucilage-(noun), a complex sticky carbohydrate secreted by certain plants that protects mucosal membranes and inflamed tissue

Mucolytic- (adjective), mucus dissolving

Mucosa- (noun), mucous membrane

Mucosal membrane- (noun), tissue that lines all entrances to the human body

Mucus- (noun), thick, slimy fluid secreted by mucosal membranes

Naturopathy- a system of medicine that uses herbs and other natural methods to stimulate the body to heal itself without the use of synthetic drugs

Necrosis- (noun), the death of cells in an organ or tissue

Neoplasia- (noun), a tumor

Nephralgia- (noun), pain in the renal (kidney) or loin area

Nephritis- (noun), an inflammation of the kidney

Nervine herb- (adjective + noun), an herb that calms the nervous system, acting as a sedative

Neuralgia- (noun), pain from irritation or inflammation of nerves

Neuritis- (noun), inflammation of nerves

Neuropathy- (noun), neuritis

Neurotransmitters- (noun), chemicals that transmit nerve impulses

Night sweats- (noun), copious quantities of perspiration while sleeping

Nocturia- (noun), the need to pass urine at night, interfering with sleep

Nutritive herb- (adjective + noun), an herb that provides food value

Occlusion- (noun), the closing of an organ or body part

Officinal- (adjective), from the Latin *officinalis*, relating to an herb species with medicinal value

OTC- (adjective), over the counter; medication available without prescription

Oxytocic- (adjective), induces uterine contractions

Palliative- (adjective), medicine that relieves symptoms but does not cure the disease

Palpitation- (noun), an abnormal heartbeat

Papule- (noun), a small, superficial spot on the skin

Parasite- (noun), an organism that lives in another living organism while making no useful contribution to the host

Parasympathetic nervous system- (noun), that part of the nervous system involved in vegetative functions, eg. digestion

Parturient- (adjective), aiding childbirth

Pathogen- (noun), a microorganism that causes disease

Pathogenic- (adjective), causing or producing disease

Pectoral- (adjective), acting on the lungs

Peptic ulcer- (noun), collectively referring to gastric and duodenal ulcers

Peptide- (noun), a compound protein with two or more amino acids

Pericarditis- (noun), an inflammation of the outside lining of the heart

Periodontal disease- (noun), a disease of the gums

Peripheral circulation- (noun), blood supply to the periphery of the body: the limbs, skin and muscle

Peripheral- (adjective), pertaining to the surface or outside

Peripheral resistance- (noun), opposition to flood flow

Peristalsis- (verb), involuntary muscle contractions in the digestive tract that moves its contents along

Peritonitis- (noun), an inflammation of the abdominal cavity

PH- (noun), a scale ranging from 0-14 measuring acidity; 7 is neutral

Pharmacopoeia- (noun), an official compendium of drugs in use for each given country

Pharyngitis- (noun), inflammation of the pharynx; sore throat

Phenol- (noun), an aromatic compound with a hydroxy group (-OH), hanging on it

Phlebitis- (noun) an inflammation of the wall of a vein

Phlegm- (noun), a thick mucus secreted by the walls of the respiratory tract; sputum; loogey

Photosensitivity- (noun), extreme sensitivity to sun and light

Physic- (noun), a laxative; cathartic

Phytoestrogens- (noun), plant compounds with estrogenic effects

Phytohormones- (noun), plant compounds that mimic human hormones

Phytotherapy- (noun), treatment of disease by plants; herbal medicine

Piles- (noun), hemorrhoids

Placebo- (noun), a fake dose used in clinical trials

Plasma- (noun), the fluid portion of the blood that cells float in

Pleurisy- (noun), an inflammation of the covering of the lungs

Pneumonia- (noun), an infection of the lungs

Pneumothorax- (noun), a collapsed lung

Polyp- (noun), a benign growth on mucosal membrane

Polysaccharide- (noun), a molecule composed of many sugars linked together

Poultice- (noun), a compress

Prognosis- (noun), a prediction of the future course of outcome of a disease

Prophylactic- (adjective), preventative

Prostaglandin- (noun), a short-term hormone-like substance

Prostatitis- (noun), inflammation of the prostate gland

Prostration- (noun), complete exhaustion

Protease- (noun), a protein-cleaving enzyme

Protein- (noun), an organic substance containing amino acids

Pruritis- (noun), itching

Psoriasis- (noun), a chronic skin condition, characterized by itchy, scaly patches

Pulmonary embolism- (noun), normally, a blood clot blocking blood supply in the lung

Pungent- (adjective), sharp or biting in taste or odor

Purgative- (noun), a strong laxative

Pus- (noun), a thick light yellow to greenish liquid containing blood and dead cells

Pustule- (noun), pus-containing blister

Putrefaction- (noun), rotting

Pyorrhea- (noun), gum disease

Qi- (noun), Chi, syn: vital energy force in Chinese philosophy

REM sleep- (noun), dream sleep

Renal calculus- (noun), a kidney stone

Renin- (noun), an enzyme secreted by the kidneys

Resin- (noun), a plant exudate with semi-solid viscous principles

Respiration- (noun), the exchange of gasses, i.e. oxygen and carbon dioxide, between the body tissues and the environment

Restorative- (adjective), revives health of strength

Reye's syndrome- (noun), swelling of the brain and affected organ due to the use of aspirin during certain viral infections (flu, chicken pox), typically in children

Rheumatism- (noun), a loose term meaning any disorder causing aches and pains in muscles or joints

Rheumatoid arthritis- (noun), an autoimmune disease that attacks joints

Rhizome- (noun), a creeping horizontal stem sitting just on, or just under the ground's surface

Rosacea- (noun), chronic acne around the nose, forehead, and cheeks

Rubefacient- (noun), a substance that causes redness of the skin, increases blood flow, and facilitates cleansing of tissue

Saccharide- (noun), a sugar molecule

Saponins- (noun), a group of soap-like glycosides found in some plants that have physiologic effects on the body, some of which are steroid-like

Scabies- (noun), an infection caused by mite infestation

Sciatica- (noun), shooting pain down the back of thigh usually due to disc disintegration

Sclerosis- (noun), a process of scarring or hardening

Seborrhea- (noun), excess secretion of the sebaceous glands

Secretion- (noun), synthesis and release of a substance by a cell or organ

Sedative- (adjective), reduces tension, calming

Senile dementia- (noun), mental deterioration associated with the aging process

Septicemia- (noun), tissue destruction caused by pathogenic bacteria or toxins absorbed from the bloodstream; blood poisoning

Serum- (noun), what is left of the blood when all cells are removed

Shingles- (noun), a viral infection of the nerves caused by the herpes virus; herpes zoster

Sialogogue- (noun), a substance that stimulates the secretion of saliva

Soporific- (noun), a substance that induces sleep

Spasmolytic- (noun) a substance that relaxes muscles

Species- (noun), the basic unit of plant classification under genus

Sprue- (noun), malabsorption due to intestinal disease

Sputum- (noun), phlegm

Stenosis- (noun), abnormal narrowing of blood vessels or heart valves

Steroids- (noun) compounds with a characteristic ring structure that make up sex and adrenal hormones

Sterol- (noun), a waxy, steroid alcohol, like cholesterol

Stimulant- (noun) a substance that increases activity

Stomachic- (noun), a substance that eases stomach pain or increases stomach activity, and aids digestion and appetite

Stroke- (noun), sudden loss of consciousness followed by paralysis caused by hemorrhage into the brain, formation of an embolism that blocks an artery, or rupture of an artery causing hemorrhage

Sty- (noun), a bacterial infection of a gland at the base of an eyelash

Styptic- (noun), a substance that stops bleeding

Sudorific- (noun), a substance that causes sweating

Surfactant- (noun), a substance that reduces the surface tension of water; a soap; a substance that allows oily and non-oily substances to be combined

Sycosis- (noun), inflammation of hair follicles

Sympathetic nervous system- (noun), that part of the nervous system involved in arousal, alertness, and muscle tone

Sympatholytic herb- (noun), an herb that down-regulates the sympathetic nervous system

Synapse- (noun), a junction between nerve cells

Syncope- (noun), fainting due to a loss of blood to the brain

Syndrome- (noun), group of symptoms that occur together characteristic of a particular disorder

Systemic- (adjective), affecting the whole body rather than individual tissues

Tachypenea- (noun), rapid breathing

Tannins- (noun), compounds that react with proteins to produce a leather-like coating on animal tissue; promote healing and numbing; reduce inflammation

Tendonitis- (noun), an inflammation the fibers that connect muscle to bone and joints

Terpene- (noun), an active plant component with a carbon ring structure, generally highly aromatic and found in volatile oils

Thrombotic- (adjective), blood clot forming

Tincture- (noun), an alcohol, or water and alcohol, herbal solution

Tinnitis- (noun), a subjective ringing in the ear

Tissue- (noun), a group of similar cells that perform a particular function

Tone- (verb), to strengthen or restore

Tonic- (noun), a substance that increases the functional tone of either a single organ or the entire body; nurtures and enlivens

Topical- (adjective), applied to surface of body

Toxemia- (noun), accumulation of toxins in the blood

Toxic- (adjective), harmful or poisonous

Toxin- (noun), a poisonous substance

Ulcerative colitis- (noun), inflammation and ulceration of the lower gastrointestinal tract

Urea- (noun), nitrogen waste product of the kidney

Urethritis- (noun), inflammation of the urethra

Urticaria- (noun), hives

Vaginitis- (noun), inflammation of the vagina usually due to infection

Varicose veins- (noun), distended veins in the legs or rectum (hemorrhoids) due to congestion

Vasoconstriction- (noun), a narrowing of the walls or blood vessels

Vasodilatation- (noun), a relaxing of the walls of blood vessels

Vermifuge- (noun), a substance that destroys and expels intestinal worms

Vertigo- (noun), dizziness; feeling of one's surroundings being in motion

Vesicant- (noun), a substance that causes blistering to the skin; counterirritant

Virulent- (adjective), having the ability to produce disease

Virus- (noun), a disease-causing microorganism capable of replicating only in living cells

Volatile oils- (noun), a complex mixture of organic compounds that evaporate when exposed to air; usually the odiferous components of plants

Vulnerary- (adjective), applied topically (externally) to enhance wound healing

Warming remedy- (noun), usually spicy, pungent herbs that dispel coldness, and stimulate circulation and digestion

Wart- (noun), a small hard growth caused by a virus

Xerostomia- (noun), reduced saliva causing dry mouth

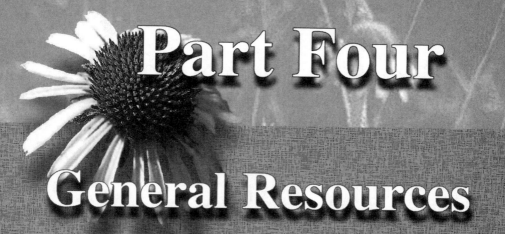

Part Four

General Resources

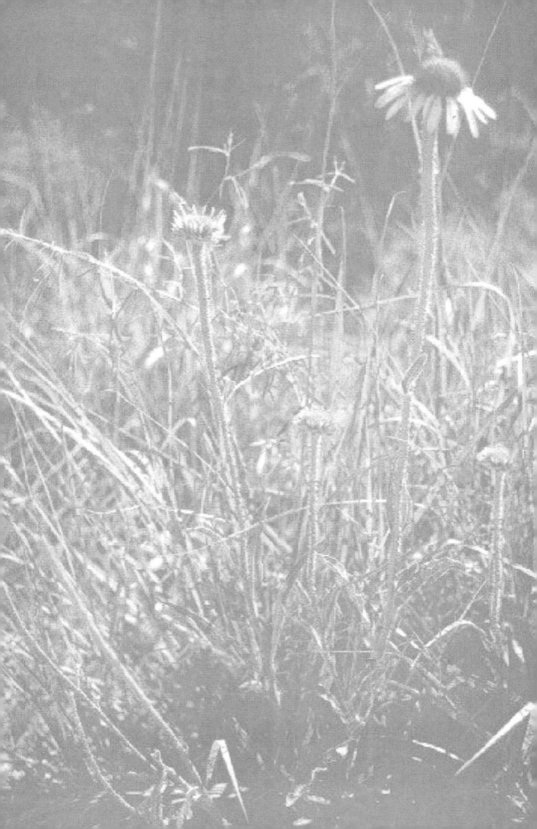

General Bibliography

Bartram, T. *Encyclopedia of Herbal Medicine*. Christchurch, England. Grace Publishers. 1995.

Bensky, D, et al. *Chinese Herbal Medicine: Materia Medica*. Seattle, WA. Eastland Press. 1993.

Bisset, N. *Herbal Drugs and Phytopharmaceuticals*. London, England. CRC Press. 1994.

Blumenthal M. et al. *The Complete German Commission E Monographs - Therapeutic Guide to Herbal Medicines*. Austin, TX. American Botanical Council. 1998.

Blumenthal, M, et al. *Herbal Medicine – Expanded Commission E Monographs*. Newton, MA. Integrative Medicine Communications. 2000.

Blumenthal, M, Riggins, C. *Popular Herbs in the U.S. Market, Therapeutic Monographs*, Austin, TX: American Botanical Council. 1997.

Boik, J. *Cancer & Natural Medicine*. Princeton, MN. Oregon Medical Press. 1996.

Bradley, P. ed. *British Herbal Compendium*. Bournemouth, England. British Herbal Medicine Association. 1992.

Bown, D. *Encyclopedia of Herbs & Their Uses*. New York, NY. Dorling Kindersley Publishing. 1995.

Brinker, F. *Herb Contraindications and Drug Interactions*. 2nd Ed. Sandy, OR. Eclectic Medical Publications. 1998.

Bruneton, J. *Pharmacognosy, Phytochemistry, Medicinal Plants*. Andover, Hampshire. UK. Intercept Ltd. 1995.

Brown, DJ. *Herbal Prescriptions for Better Health*. Rocklin, CA. Prima Publishing. 1996.

Chevallier A. *Encyclopedia of Medicinal Plants*. New York: DK Publishing. 1996.

Christopher, D. director. *The School of Natural Healing: 100 Herb Syllabus*. Springville, UT. 1996.

Crellin, J and Philpott, J. *A Reference Guide to Medicinal Plants*. Durham and London, England. Duke University Press. 1990.

Duke, J. *The Green Pharmacy*. Emmaus, PA. Rodale Press. 1997.

Foster, S, Tyler, V. *Tyler's Honest Herbal*. New York/London. The Haworth Herbal Press. 1999.

Gordon, R. *The Alarming History of Medicine*. NY, NY. St. Martin's Press. 1993.

Griggs, B. *Green Pharmacy*. Rochester, VE. Healing Arts Press. 1991.

Grieve, M. *A Modern Herbal*. New York, NY. Dover Publications. 1971.

Gruenwald, J, et al, eds. *PDR for Herbal Medicines*. Montvale, NJ. Medical Economics Company, Inc. 1998.

Hoffmann, D. *The Herbalist* CD-ROM Ver. 2.0. Hopkins, MN. Topkins Technology 1992.

Huang, K. *The Pharmacology of Chinese Herbs*. Boca Raton, FL. CRC Press. 1999.

Jellin, J, et al. *Natural Medicines Comprehensive Database*. Stockton, CA. Therapeutic Research Faculty. 1999.

Li, T. *Medicinal Plants*. Lancanster, PA. Technomic Publishing Company. 2000.

McGuffin, M. et al. *American Herbal Products Association's Botanical Safety Book*. Boca Raton, FL. CRC Press. 1997.

Moss, R. *Herbs Against Cancer*. Brooklyn, NY. Equinox Press. 1998.

Mowrey D. *The Scientific Validation of Herbal Medicine*. New Canaan, Connecticut. Keats Publ. 1986.

Mowrey D. *Guaranteed Potency Herbs; Next Generation Herbal Medicine*. New Canaan, Connecticut. Keats Publ. 1990.

Newall, C, et al. *Herbal Medicines. A Guide for Health-Care Professionals*. London, England. Pharmaceutical Press. 1998.

Ody, P. *The Complete Medicinal Herbal*. New York, NY. Dorling Kindersley. 1993.

Pedersen, M. *Nutritional Herbology*. Warsaw, IN. Wendell W. Whitman Company, 1995.

Rister, R. *Japanese Herbal Medicine*. Garden City, NY. Avery Publishing Group. 1999.

Robbers, J. et al. *Pharmacognosy and Pharmacobiotechnology*. Baltimore, MA. Williams & Wilkins. 1996.

Schulz, V, et al. *Rational Phytotherapy: A Physician's Guide to Herbal Medicine*. Berlin. Springer-Verlag. 1998

Weiss R. *Herbal Medicine*. Beaconsfield, England: Beaconsfield Publ. Ltd. 1988.

Wetton, P, et al. *British Herbal Pharmacopoeia*. Bournemouth, England. British Herbal Medicine Association. 1996.

Zhu, Y. *Chinese Materia Medica*. Amsterdam, Netherlands. Harwood Academic Publishers. 1998.

Index